BASALT REGIONAL

99 MIDLAND AVENUE
BASALT CO 81621
927-4311

D1533259

618.2 GRO
Groenou, Aneema van.
The active woman's guide to
$16.95
06/04

OCT 1 8 2004	DATE DUE	

The **Active Woman's** Guide to **Pregnancy**

Practical Advice for **Getting Outdoors** When Expecting

Aneema Van Groenou, M.D.

BASALT REGIONAL LIBRARY
99 MIDLAND AVENUE
BASALT CO 81621-8305

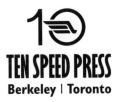

TEN SPEED PRESS
Berkeley | Toronto

For the lively, fit, and enlightened

pregnant adventurers whose appreciation

of the outdoors can make this world a

better place for generations to come.

Copyright © 2004 by Aneema Van Groenou
Front cover photography © 2003 by Jonathan Chester
Photograph on page xii by Thinkstock/Getty Images
Photograph on page 14 by Adam Crowley/Getty Images
Photograph on page 28 by Sergio Knaebel
Photograph on page 40 by Photodisc Blue/Getty Images
Photograph on page 52 by Jonathan Chester
Photograph on page 66 by Ryan McVay/Getty Images
Photograph on page 72 by Jules Frazier/Getty Images
Photograph on page 82 by Photodisc Blue/Getty Images
Photograph on page 132 by Photodisc Blue/Getty Images
Photograph on page 168 by Thinkstock/ Getty Images
Photograph on page 228 by Photodisc Blue/Getty Images
Photograph on page 272 by Photodisc Blue/ Getty Images

All rights reserved. No part of this book may be
reproduced in any form, except brief excerpts for
the purpose of review, without written permission
of the publisher.

A Kirsty Melville Book

Ten Speed Press
Box 7123
Berkeley, California 94707
www.tenspeed.com

Distributed in Australia by Simon and Schuster
Australia, in Canada by Ten Speed Press Canada, in
New Zealand by Southern Publishers Group, in South
Africa by Real Books, and in the United Kingdom and
Europe by Airlift Book Company.

Design by Catherine Jacobes Design

Library of Congress Cataloging-in-Publication Data

Van Groenou, Aneema.
The active woman's guide to pregnancy : practical
advice for getting outdoors when expecting / Aneema
Van Groenou.
        p. cm.
"A Kirsty Melville Book."
Includes bibliographical references and index.
ISBN 1-58008-518-0 (pbk.)
    1. Exercise for pregnant women. 2. Outdoor
recreation. I. Title.
    RG558.7 .G76   2004
    618.2'44—dc22   2003017867

Printed in the United States of America
First printing, 2004

1 2 3 4 5 6 7 8 9 10 — 08 07 06 05 04

Contents

Acknowledgments

I'd like to extend my thanks to the many people who shared my enthusiasm for this project and helped this book come alive. Special thanks to my pregnant muses, especially to Kate Hackett, Jennifer Hayes, Jen Kramer Tate, Dr. Carrie Mendoza, Emily Odelberg, Stacy Waterman-Hoey, Susan Ward Coffey, Dr. Kati Watt, and to the many women who filled out questionnaires with tales of expectant adventure. For support in the writing process, thanks to Dr. Peter Hackett, Dr. Paul Auerbach, Dr. Lee Shockley, and Meimei Fox. Thanks to the outdoor adventurers Diana Bermudez, Will Hildesley, and Jen Hayes for lending a critical eye to the fledgling manuscript. I am very grateful to my agent, Felicia Eth, for being my advocate; to my editors, Holly Taines White, for her keen and appropriately pregnant insight; and Carrie Rodrigues, for her attention to detail and sense of style; and to my publisher, Kirsty Melville at Ten Speed, for taking up this project. This book took wing because of the gifts from my family, Willem, Meher, and Saleem Van Groenou: of the love of teaching and of recognizing the essential nature of playing outdoors. Sergio Knaebel, for all the happy trails: thank you.

Introduction

Only fifty years ago, being pregnant meant staying off your feet, avoiding robust activity, and even being treated as if you were ill. But for most women today, the thought of giving up their active lifestyles for nine months or more is distressing—and seems unhealthy. And they're right. Finally, medical research has caught up with the convictions of these spirited women (and there are a lot of us out there!) and proven that regular exercise during pregnancy has many real benefits, from less back pain to a shorter labor. Exercise doesn't wear out your pregnant body; it conditions it. Staying active will help you have a healthier pregnancy, delivery, and baby—and a more positive outlook. So even before you feel that first kick inside your belly, here's a gentle kick in the pants to get out there and stay active!

I have written this book to encourage you to continue the outdoor activities you enjoy the most—not only because they are good for your pregnancy but also because they are good for you. For many women, activities like running, gardening, and kayaking are great ways to stay in shape, spend time with loved ones, enjoy the outdoors, and gather some peace of mind. If you want to bike around the neighborhood or swim in the local pool, go for it. If you are a bit more adventurous and prefer hiking and snowshoeing, don't give them up. You will be surprised to learn how much you can do during pregnancy. In this book, I will help you plan and modify your activities so that they are safe for you and your baby. I recommend that you be cautious—but also do what's fun for you. Ask yourself: what do I *feel* like going out and doing today?

This is the first pregnancy book that helps you choose your own activities instead of requiring you to adapt your lifestyle to somebody else's exercise regimen. This is your nuts-and-bolts adviser on how to nurture a healthy pregnancy while staying active—and it's loaded with tips on how to plan ahead, what to watch out for, what to take with you, and what to expect. I have brought together all the latest medical research on exercise as it relates to pregnancy so that you can understand the real benefits and risks and get beyond the many myths about what you can and can't do.

Use the book however you like. You don't have to read it straight through or get hung up on the medical information. If you're short on time, you can just flip to the activity you're interested in and get the facts you need to enjoy a healthy excursion. Keep this book handy for use as a quick reference—and a source of inspiration.

You know your body best, so take care to listen to your body and slow down when you need to. Pay close attention to my recommendations about the risk for each activity: low (good for beginners), medium (possible for experienced and confident athletes), or high (not recommended, even for highly trained athletes) each trimester. Before starting an exercise regimen talk with your doctor about any special circumstances that may affect the exercises you can do safely. Find a doctor you feel comfortable with and ask a lot of questions; every pregnancy is different and no book will address all your individual concerns about pregnancy or exercise.

Every activity in this book will help you stay strong and fit while getting some fresh air. If you didn't exercise before pregnancy, start slow and don't give up because you break a sweat after three minutes or feel short of breath after five; this is normal—and worth it. If you exercise now, you're getting your pregnancy started on the right foot and will reap the rewards of a healthy lifestyle for years to come.

Congratulations! Just by picking up this book, you are taking the first step toward having an active pregnancy and giving your baby the healthiest possible start in life.

What do you feel like going out and doing?	Try one of these:
I want to stay fit during pregnancy.	☐ Swimming ☐ Paddling ☐ Running ☐ Biking
I want to try something new during pregnancy.	☐ Snorkeling ☐ Camping ☐ Cross-country skiing ☐ Kayaking ☐ Snowshoeing
Oops! I'm halfway through pregnancy and I haven't exercised yet; I want to get started.	☐ Swimming ☐ Walking ☐ Cross-country skiing ☐ Biking
I want to do something to beat the third trimester blues.	☐ Gardening ☐ Walking ☐ Canoeing ☐ Camping ☐ Snowshoeing
I need some peace and quiet. What can I do?	☐ Hiking ☐ Boating ☐ Snowshoeing ☐ Mountain biking ☐ Camping
I want to take my kids with me when I exercise.	☐ Hiking ☐ Gardening ☐ Canoeing ☐ Biking
I don't have a lot of time to get outdoors; what exercise can I fit into my tight schedule?	☐ Running ☐ Biking ☐ Gardening ☐ Walking

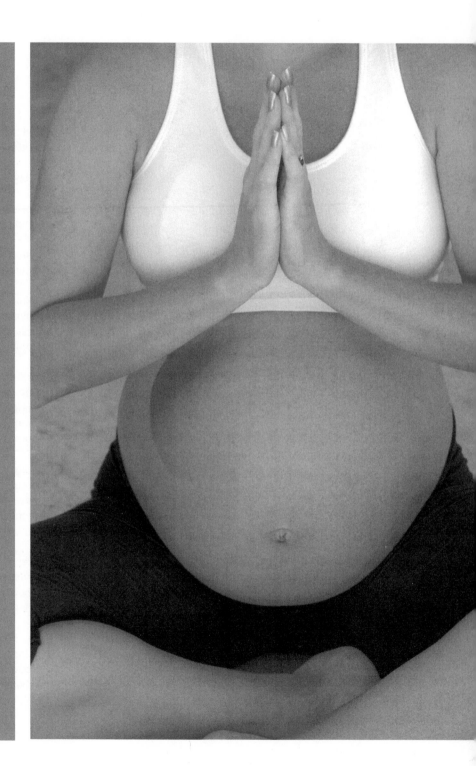

Benefits of
Staying Active

One of the best things about staying active during pregnancy is that you feel great. As many studies have shown—and active moms will tell you—if you maintain a regular exercise regimen, your body will be in better shape throughout pregnancy and more fit for delivery. For most pregnant women, exercising regularly has measurable results: less fatigue, less back pain, less moodiness, less incontinence, an easier delivery, and a quicker post-delivery recovery. And don't forget the stress relief and sheer fun of spending time outdoors!

Exercise has real payoffs for your fetus as well, such as fewer required medical interventions at birth and better weight and intelligence profiles long after birth. Believe it or not, your exercising during pregnancy may even help your baby establish a healthy lifestyle down the road.

Your exercise goals may not be very different than they were before pregnancy. But if you've always focused on competing or losing weight, you will have to change your outlook. Becoming familiar with the advantages of prenatal exercise will help you set goals that feel good for you *and* benefit your pregnancy.

How much and how often you exercise is up to you. As was the case before you became pregnant, consistency is key to staying fit. A typical healthy schedule involves exercising at least thirty minutes per day, three times a week. You'll find that outdoor activities are more flexible; you may hike for an hour and a half one day, jog for fifteen minutes the next, and spend an entire Saturday morning working in the garden. Thinking about your goals won't banish that delicious flexibility; it will simply help you incorporate activities specifically for their pregnancy benefits.

Some of the most valuable rewards of regular exercise are less tangible. Spending time outside—with your partner, friends, or dog—may help you catch your breath and gain some perspective on all the changes in your life. If you spend this relaxed time with loved ones, you will also strengthen your relationships and develop some of the good communication and support you will depend on after delivery.

chapter 1

Staying Active for Total-Body Fitness

Staying active during pregnancy keeps you fit. This means your heart and lungs work more efficiently, your muscles and bones stay stronger, and your hormones stabilize your blood sugar levels more effectively. But what you will really notice when you exercise regularly is that you eventually feel less tired and less achy (and maybe more cheerful). You may also notice that you leak less urine when coughing and have fewer varicose veins. From your breathing to your bones, exercise pays off for you and your baby-soon-to-be-born.

A Fit Heart. Your heart is a muscle that is working out all the time, delivering oxygen and nutrients to your body. During pregnancy, your heart works even harder, beating faster and pumping more blood than before you were pregnant, sending all those nutrients and oxygen to your growing body and your growing fetus. The heart literally becomes bigger (the left ventricle dilates to hold more blood and the muscular wall thickens). By the end of the second trimester, your heart pumps 40 to 50 percent more blood per minute than before pregnancy—and this is while you are resting!

Exercising also increases your total volume of blood, but luckily it does not increase your risk of anemia or low blood iron. Fit women are able to exercise harder during pregnancy because their hearts can pump more blood while maintaining a lower heart rate. You can build your stamina—or cardiovascular fitness—by regularly doing *aerobic* activities that work your heart, lungs, and large muscle groups, such as walking, running, swimming, hiking, paddling, and biking. If you want to build stamina, set a regular exercise schedule and choose an activity you'll stick with.

Healthy Lungs. If you exercise regularly, you will find that your lungs become more fit—just like your heart and other muscles do. Your lungs provide oxygen for you and for your developing fetus: it's not an easy task, since the growing pregnancy puts upward pressure on the diaphragm and makes breathing deeply more and more difficult. It may feel like you can't get enough air sometimes, but your normal resting breaths (called *tidal volume*) are not affected by your growing belly.

When you exercise, your lungs work even harder to supply the pumping heart and muscles. You will notice that you become short of breath more easily with exertion, especially as the pregnancy progresses. But, with regular exercise, your lungs will become conditioned to deliver more oxygen to your blood and body, so you won't become short of breath as quickly.

Better Sugar Control. Regular, moderate exercise during pregnancy can also help to control your blood sugar level. Women who exercise regularly are less likely to develop diabetes, an illness in which the blood sugar is not well regulated. Diabetes can cause problems during pregnancy such as increased birth weight and difficult delivery. The greatly fluctuating sugar level in uncontrolled diabetes can also harm the fetus, causing birth defects and even death.

Women who already have diabetes or who develop gestational diabetes (pregnancy-related diabetes) are advised to exercise, change their diet, and get medical treatment, to help control their blood sugar level.

Even if you don't have diabetes, exercise helps your body become more sensitive to insulin, the hormone that regulates the body's sugar level. Studies have shown that exercise that uses large muscle groups (such as aerobic exercises like walking, running, swimming, and cross-country skiing) improves muscles' responsiveness so your blood sugar is better regulated. Regular exercise—with regular snacks—may help you both prevent and treat sugar imbalances.

Feel-Good Endorphins. You may already know that exercise stimulates the release of chemicals in the brain that produce a feeling of well-being. You have probably experienced this effect when working out gave you a burst of energy or walking around the block improved your mood. These chemicals, called *endorphins*, function like opiates such as morphine. They can minimize pain and improve your sleep. When you exercise this natural chemical response makes you feel more relaxed.

Regular exercise may also stimulate the release of more endorphins during labor and delivery, when you really need them. One study reviewed by the *Journal of Perinatal Medicine* showed that regular exercisers had higher endorphin levels at delivery and experienced less pain during labor.

Good Posture. As your pregnancy grows, your skeletal system—your bones and ligaments—adjusts to your body's new center of gravity. The uterus itself grows up to a thousand times its nonpregnant volume. Your breasts grow too and can each weigh over a pound (five hundred grams) extra at term. This increased weight and your altered shape change the way you carry your body.

The protuberant belly, the arched back (called *lordosis*), and the waddling walk are all characteristic of pregnancy. In fact, these changes are adaptations that help you maintain your balance by shifting your center of gravity backward, so you don't fall forward onto your precious belly. In order to allow for these postural changes, your body gets an influx of hormones that cause your ligaments and joints to relax. This extra flexibility also allows the baby to pass through the narrow pelvis during delivery.

Although being active during pregnancy can be more challenging because of this shift in posture, exercise can help ease some of the discomfort caused by these changes. For example, the ligament strain and discomfort in your lower back and pelvis, caused by the increased arch in your back, can be reduced significantly with regular exercise and stretching to strenghen your back muscles. Research presented in the journal *Clinics in Sports Medicine* indicates that pregnant women who do regular, moderate exercise report less back and pelvic discomfort throughout pregnancy.

Exercise may also help you become more comfortable maneuvering with your pregnant body and be better able to maintain your balance, preventing falls.

Stronger Bones. During pregnancy and breastfeeding, your hormones fluctuate and affect your calcium level and bone development. Until the last few weeks of pregnancy, the total calcium level in your blood actually drops. However, this does not affect your bone strength. Several hormonal changes compensate for the decreased calcium to maintain a relatively constant level of calcium for your own skeleton and your growing fetus's bones. And this is fortunate, since your body is building bone almost twice as fast as when you were not pregnant.

Exercises that require your bones—like your legs and spine—to bear weight help strengthen those bones, improve posture, and prevent fractures.

Weight-bearing activities, such as running, hiking, and snowshoeing, help build strong bones.

During breastfeeding, a woman's estrogen levels drop very low (as they do after menopause) and this causes bones to start losing some of their strength. Most women lose 3 to 5 percent of their bone density during the first ten to eighteen weeks of breastfeeding.

The best way to keep your bones healthy is to exercise regularly before pregnancy to build strong bones; make sure you are getting enough calcium through your diet or supplements both during and after pregnancy; and continue exercise after pregnancy to rebuild your bone strength.

Toned Muscles. As you would expect, exercise during pregnancy helps you maintain muscle tone. For many women, this means feeling good about their changing bodies. Better muscle tone means better muscular support for your bones and ligaments, so you experience fewer aches. Maintaining toned muscles also helps you get back in shape after delivery: women who exercise regularly during pregnancy regain their abdominal muscle tone after delivery more quickly than non-exercisers do. When you exercise, you also build muscles that you may not even notice, like the pelvic floor muscles. These muscles are key to pushing effectively during a vaginal delivery—and good muscle tone and flexibility may make your labor less strenuous. Many outdoor activities help develop your muscle strength and endurance. If you want to build muscle, choose activities in which you work against some resistance, such as swimming, kayaking, surfing, biking uphill, or cross-country skiing.

Better Bladder Control. One of the annoying side effects of pregnancy is the feeling of needing to urinate all the time. Many women leak urine (called *incontinence*), especially when laughing, coughing, or changing position. This incontinence is caused by the uterus putting direct pressure on the bladder, creating a feeling of urgency, and the stretching of the muscles around the vagina and urethra (where urine flows out), weakening urine control. Any activity that increases pressure in the belly, such as lifting something heavy, can cause urine leakage during pregnancy. Certainly, as your pregnancy progresses, you should be prepared to stop any activity frequently to urinate.

Women who exercise regularly recover their normal bladder control more quickly after giving birth. According to studies done by Dr. James Clapp, a renowned obstetric exercise researcher, only 20 percent of exercising women still experience incontinence one year after delivery, versus 42 percent of non-exercising women. Regular exercise seems to alleviate, rather than aggravate, bladder control problems during and after pregnancy.

Fewer Varicose Veins and Blood Clots. Your high hormone levels and greater body weight increase your chances of developing varicose veins and blood clots during pregnancy. However, moderate exercise such as walking and swimming can help prevent varicose veins by improving circulation and helping to stimulate the muscles in the legs, causing the blood to return to the heart, rather than pool in the veins.

In some cases, high-impact activities such as running may make larger varicose veins more obvious—but only temporarily. Also, standing for long periods increases the pressure in the veins; elevating your legs and feet above the level of your heart or wearing support stockings will help reduce the swelling. Remember that most varicose veins will resolve slowly after delivery.

Blood clots (also called *deep vein thrombosis*), which are more common during pregnancy, pose a serious risk since they can travel to the lungs via the bloodstream and become life threatening. Regular exercise, even gentle activity, helps maintain good circulation and can help prevent blood clots. If you are sitting for long periods—such as on a plane or in a car—doing a little light exercise, such as walking, for a few minutes every hour can dramatically reduce your risk.

Less Painful Labor. One excellent reason to stay in shape during pregnancy is that exercise prepares you so well for a strenuous labor. Fit mothers know that their physical conditioning made delivery easier—and studies show that they are right on target.

Several studies reviewed in the *American Journal of Obstetrics and Gynecology* have shown that fit women who deliver vaginally labor for less time. In one study, women who were physically fit tended to complete the dilation phase of labor (during which the cervix opens) in an average of four hours versus six hours for the non-exercisers. Also, the pushing stage (which lasts through when the baby is born) took the exercisers, on average, thirty-six minutes and the non-exercisers sixty minutes.

Women who exercise also say they experience less pain during labor. In several studies, fit women reported less pain during labor and asked for less pain medication than non-exercisers did. In one study, women who had engaged in endurance exercise during pregnancy needed epidural anesthesia for pain control during delivery in only 28 percent of deliveries versus in 50 percent of non-exercising women's births.

Labor tends to start a few days earlier—but still at term—for exercising women. A majority of exercisers deliver before their due date. In contrast, half of non-exercising women deliver after theirs.

Quicker Post-Pregnancy Recovery. Women who exercise during pregnancy tend to recover more quickly and are more likely to return to their pre-pregnancy levels of fitness after delivery.

According to research by Dr. Clapp, over 90 percent of the women who exercised during pregnancy continue to exercise after delivery. And most of these women (70 percent) are in better shape a year after delivery than they were before they got pregnant!

Most fit women start exercising again two weeks after a vaginal delivery (or a little longer after a cesarean section)—but you may find that your own recovery time ranges from three days to eight weeks.

Good Weight Management. Don't think of exercise as a way to control your weight during pregnancy—healthy weight gain is a very important part of supporting your growing fetus. Further, fat helps in the production of essential hormones for pregnancy, and it efficiently stores energy for you and your fetus.

Try to follow your doctor's recommended guidelines for weight gain, typically twenty-five to thirty-five pounds. Exercise can help you in this endeavor, preventing excessive weight gain, especially extra fat in the late second and third trimesters.

Keep in mind that exercising during and after your pregnancy does not necessarily mean that you will lose your pregnancy weight quickly. For most women, whether they exercise or not, weight loss after delivery is gradual, since you need to eat more while breastfeeding. In the long run, however, women who exercise are 30 percent more likely to return to their pre-pregnancy fat and weight levels within a year of delivery—and continue a healthy lifestyle that will keep them fit down the road.

A fitness regimen for maintaining a healthy weight involves a mix of aerobic exercises, such as hiking and swimming, and muscle-building exercises, such as mountain biking and snowshoeing. Depending on the season, you can meet your fitness goals by combining outdoor activities with a gym workout or prenatal exercise class, for a minimum of one and one-half hours per week.

Staying Active for Fun

Women take up an active lifestyle for many reasons—weight control, long-term health benefits, preparing for delivery—but they keep it up because they really enjoy it. You may find that spending time outside allows you to collect your thoughts, walk off the stresses of the day, get away from the tasks and tensions of your household, and spend some valuable time with loved ones. Listed below are some of the best reasons to head outdoors during pregnancy.

A Positive Emotional Outlook. In many ways, exercise—particularly outdoor exercise—contributes to your sense of well-being during pregnancy. Since outdoor activities often take you to inspiring natural locations and allow you to spend time with friends, you may appreciate a healthy sense of balance and joy in your life. In fact, on psychiatric questionnaires women who exercise regularly during pregnancy report 60 percent fewer symptoms of depression than non-exercisers.

Stress Relief. When you are pregnant, you need every break you can get from the stress of planning and preparing for your baby's arrival. Fitting in a stroll around the block does a good deal more than give you a short breather.

Exercise may relieve stress in many ways, including improving sleep, making personal time for unwinding and reflection, and increasing levels of natural relaxants in the body. Not surprisingly, according to an article in the journal *Clinics in Sports Medicine*, women who exercise regularly enjoy a more relaxed mother-child relationship than non-exercisers do, one year after delivery. Try to get a little time outside every day, even if it's just fifteen minutes; your hormones respond to exposure to natural light. Also, avoid exercising within two hours of bedtime, when the elevated endorphins can interfere with your ability to fall asleep. Some women find that exercising at a consistent time of day also helps regulate mood and helps them sleep better.

Learning to Listen to Your Body. During pregnancy, your body communicates its changes with subtle signs: a blush in the cheeks, darkening of the nipples, an increased appetite. Throughout pregnancy, your body uses this language of signals to give clues about its needs and limits. Because exercise—especially outdoor exercise—involves such a variety of movements and can also provide a quiet time for introspection, it helps you to become more sensitive to your body.

The expecting woman slowly learns to recognize those signals: that ache means *slow down*, the nausea means *eat something*, that pressure means *go urinate again*. And, after a time, your baby starts speaking to you too, with gentle flutters and then outright kicks. For each of us, the signals are individual, personal. Learning to listen to your body is an important skill that you can use to be able to detect possible problems during your pregnancy and to stay safe while being active.

Good Parenting. Think that parenting doesn't start until you hear that first wail? Think again. For most couples, pregnancy is a time to establish healthy habits, get the home and finances in order, set long-term goals, and found a healthy parenting relationship. Despite all this preparation, the pregnancy can feel overwhelming, with all the doctor's appointments and tests, the changing dynamics of your relationships, the sometimes incomprehensible and annoying symptoms, and your undeniably ballooning body. Setting priorities, keeping your cool, and cultivating a positive outlook are all part of pregnancy—call it "Introduction to Parenting."

Staying Active for Your Baby

During your pregnancy, your growing fetus becomes a priority in your life. Even before your child is born, you want to give him or her the healthiest possible start in life. It's not surprising that your exercising during pregnancy benefits your fetus—improving blood flow and providing important physical stimulation. What *is* surprising is that the fetus's exposure to exercise in the womb has some long-term advantages, such as a healthier birth weight and higher intelligence.

A Healthy Placenta. The placenta is your fetus's lifeline. Your fetus depends on the placenta for receiving oxygen and nutrients from you and for removing waste from its bloodstream. Your regular exercise affects the development of the placenta in both early and mid-pregnancy. When you exercise regularly for extended periods during pregnancy, your placenta may grow bigger.

Studies presented in the journals *Placenta* and *Seminars in Perinatology* have shown that exercising women have, on average, larger placentas (by volume) and that the areas of oxygen and nutrient exchange on the placenta may also be bigger, possibly meaning that more blood flows through the placentas of fit women.

Fewer Interventions Required at Delivery. When you exercise, you may be increasing your chances of having a healthy delivery, with fewer medical interventions. Women who exercise regularly have fewer cesarean sections and forceps deliveries and need less oxytocin (a hormone used to stimulate and strengthen contractions).

Regular exercise during pregnancy makes you more likely to have an uncomplicated vaginal delivery. A study presented in the journal *Medicine and Science in Sports and Exercise* found that women who continued aerobic activities during pregnancy had better than an 85 percent chance of having a healthy vaginal delivery (called a *normal spontaneous vaginal delivery*). Women who didn't exercise or stopped exercising during pregnancy had only a 50 to 55 percent chance of having a normal spontaneous vaginal delivery. Fit women also have fewer interventions during vaginal delivery, such as use of forceps (an instrument used to grasp and deliver the baby's head). In one study, non-exercisers had forceps deliveries in 20 percent of births, while exercising women needed the assistance of forceps in just 6 percent of deliveries. Women who exercise regularly during pregnancy have fewer cesarean sections. In fact, on average, only 6 percent of exercisers have a surgical delivery, compared to 30 percent of the non-exercisers.

Dr. Clapp's studies on how endurance exercise during pregnancy affects labor show that other medical intervention during the labors of women who exercise is less common as well—such as epidural anesthesia for pain control, artificial rupture of membranes (in which a plastic hook is used to gently break the amniotic sac and stimulate labor), episiotomy (cutting the skin between the vagina and rectum to ease vaginal delivery), and intravenous hormones to stimulate regular and effective contractions. For many women, this means that regular exercise may improve your chances of having a more relaxed and natural labor and delivery.

Healthy Birth and Baby Weight. Just as you are leaner if you exercise throughout pregnancy, your baby is leaner too. After the thirty-fourth week of pregnancy (the last couple of months) is when fetuses usually gain the most fat. If the mother-to-be is exercising then, the baby is an average of seven to fourteen ounces (two hundred to four hundred grams) leaner than the baby of a non-exercising mother. This birth weight is within normal range but with less fat. These babies are just as long and their heads are just as big as the average baby. In one study, children of exercising mothers continued to be leaner at age five.

Baby's Higher Intelligence and Positive Behavior. Your exercising during pregnancy may also have some effects on your baby's behavior and intelligence. Ultrasound studies of the uterus, discussed in the journal *Seminars in Perinatology*, show that the fetus behaves differently when the mother is exercising than when she is resting. When you exercise, your fetus also participates—through the rhythmic motion, improved blood flow, vibration, higher blood sugar, and noise. This extra stimulation may affect the baby's development—even after birth.

Women who have exercised during pregnancy report that their infants are more alert, less cranky, and quiet more quickly after being disturbed. According to research presented by Dr. Clapp on neonatal behavior, newborns of exercisers orient better to sound and objects in the environment. This may mean that these babies are more developmentally advanced than the infants of less active women, even from before birth.

The advantages in behavior and intelligence in children of exercising women persist throughout childhood, as reported by the *Journal of Pediatrics*. At age one, infants of mothers who exercised during pregnancy have better motor skills. At age five, these children perform better on standardized intelligence tests, especially in oral language skills.

Staying Active for Each Other

Most things in life are easier and more fun if you do them with somebody. Pregnancy is no exception and a caring and involved partner or close friend is an important resource.

Nothing is better than sharing your thoughts with an excited partner who will support you through the pregnancy and share the joys and responsibilities even after your baby is born. Friends and other pregnant women can also be a great support. A partner or a close friend can help you stay organized, calm, prepared, and motivated. Inevitably, you'll face some enormous challenges during this pregnancy, whether in adjusting your future plans or handling a medical complication. And your life will never be the same again. Your partner faces some of the same challenges—just without the growing body. Involving your partner in caring for you and your fetus will deepen his feelings for the baby and enrich your relationship. If you are honest and open with each other, you will

How to Make Exercise Happen—Together

1. Plan ahead: make an "exercise appointment."

2. Clear your schedule: make time to warm up, exercise, and cool down.

3. Stay on track: leave distracting people, phones, pagers, and tasks behind.

4. Get good gear: change into attractive exercise clothing that makes you feel like getting outside.

5. Make it simple: choose a convenient activity and location.

6. Document your progress: it'll make you feel good about your health.

7. Have fun.

learn to appreciate each other's support and grow closer.

Pregnancy is a hectic time and the months may fly by faster than you—or your partner—can imagine. Getting outside may be one way in which you can share some valuable time together and relieve some of that stress. You will be more likely to keep up a healthy exercise routine if you do it with someone and keep each other motivated. You'll also enjoy the camaraderie of striving together to reach a common goal. Plus, you establish an important ethic: to make a healthy lifestyle a priority for your entire family.

Talk about your goals. One of your goals may be to have some time alone to unwind and listen to music. One of his goals may be to catch up with buddies during a game of hoops. That's okay. But if outdoor activities are important to both of you, set some common goals so you can enjoy them together—even during pregnancy. The point is not to add another chore to your day but to get outside for half an hour and clear your mind while energizing your body. At the same time, you'll be doing the best thing for your baby—and your relationship.

Better Communication. You may find that the time you spend outdoors is less about the exercise than about spending time with your loved ones. During evening walks, afternoon gardening sessions, rides on a ski lift, canoe trips, or hikes on the trail, you have time to share your thoughts and talk about things other than the routines and hassles of your daily life.

One of the best reasons to set common goals during pregnancy is to acknowledge the importance of making time for each other. It isn't easy now and it won't get any easier after the baby is born.

Sharing Some Fun. To many couples, outdoor activities mean exploration and adventure. Many outdoor activities will take you to places you don't see on your way to work or to the gym. You and your partner may share a love of the outdoors and pregnancy shouldn't change that one bit. Exploring a new place, whether it is a moonlit swimming pool, a hilltop view, a gleaming ski trail, or an underwater world seen through a snorkel mask, will give you some perspective. Getting outdoors arouses your curiosity and gets you out of your daily grind—so it's a true mental vacation.

Sharing outdoor activities is not only a good way to have fun with your loved ones, but it may also be safer than going out alone during pregnancy. When you are expecting, you need the support of your partner, family, and friends. Taking someone with you gives you some security in case you need help, provides an extra pair of hands to carry gear, and helps share the responsibility for taking breaks regularly.

Mutual Stress Relief. When added to the routine stress of everyday life, pregnancy—even when it is very much anticipated—can contribute to financial, family, and relationship tension. At home and at work, you may be facing ambitious goals you and your partner have decided to accomplish *before the baby comes*: getting a raise, remodeling that room, buying a new car, or spending more time with the in-laws. Getting outside can help give you some perspective on why you are excited to be parents—while relieving some of the strain that comes with preparing for this huge change in your life.

Taking your pregnancy outdoors should be as much about the fitness benefits as it is about your well-being. By staying active, you are establishing a healthy lifestyle that will reward you and your baby for a lifetime—and will prepare you well for parenting.

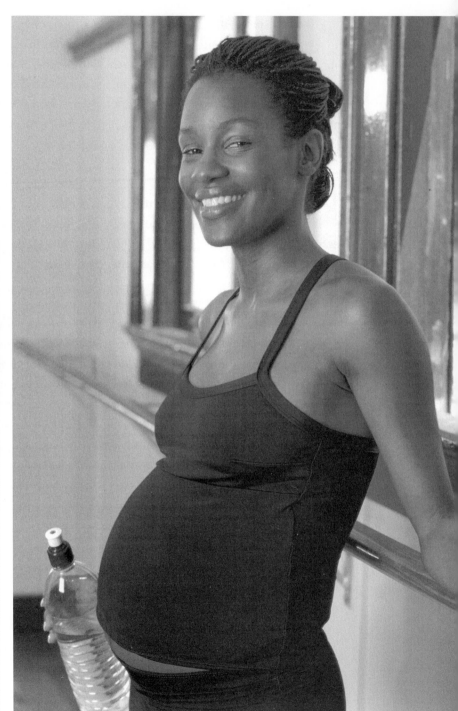

chapter

2

Q & A: WHAT ARE THE REAL
RISKS OF EXERCISE DURING
PREGNANCY?

• • •

MEDICAL EMERGENCIES

Common Concerns and Myths About Staying Active

You probably have some questions about the risks of staying active during pregnancy. That's good. Your concern will help keep you safe. If you are careful, you will be much less likely to become dehydrated, fall, or overexert yourself. Yes, these are risks with potentially dangerous consequences for the fetus—but, in reality, they are entirely preventable.

Your chances of experiencing an exercise-related problem are near zero. So why read this chapter? The more you know about how your body responds to exercise, the better prepared you are to prevent problems. Read this chapter with an eye to prevention—at each juncture, I'll tell you exactly what you can do to avoid risks.

Q & A: What Are the Real Risks of Exercise During Pregnancy?

Knowing the risks of staying active during pregnancy is important for clearing your mind—and conscience—of some common myths about exercise and pregnancy. Many misconceptions have shaped women's ideas about what is truly safe and healthy. In the last decade, a number of studies of active pregnant women have debunked the myths regarding exercise during pregnancy. So read on: getting your questions answered with the most up-to-date medical knowledge is the first step toward an active pregnancy.

Can exercise cause infertility?

No. Exercise will not cause you to become permanently sterile or make it difficult to get pregnant. Extremely rigorous levels of exercise can alter hormonal levels temporarily and inhibit ovulation. Competitive athletes, dancers, and extremely underweight women, including those with an eating disorder, may not ovulate and menstruate regularly. But as soon as they cut back on their exercise and gain some weight, their normal cycles resume. Remember that if you are menstruating, you are probably ovulating as well and can get pregnant. Chances are that you are a healthy weight and exercise moderately, so you don't have to worry that exercise will affect your chances of getting pregnant. A moderate exercise program—meaning about three to four hours a week of sweaty but not exhausting workouts—is safe and healthy even while you are trying to get pregnant.

What about causing miscarriage?

No, again. Exercising before getting pregnant and during the first trimester will not cause you to have a miscarriage. According to a study presented in the journal *Clinics in Sports Medicine*, even marathon runners who exercised well above recommended guidelines and competed in races in the first six weeks of pregnancy didn't have problems with infertility, miscarriages, birth defects, or placental problems. The healthiest things you can do when trying to conceive and during your first trimester are to quit smoking, avoid alcohol, eat well, and maintain a regular, moderate exercise schedule.

Will I be more likely to get injured if I exercise?

Not really. In fact, your chances of getting seriously hurt are about one in a hundred—just about the same as they would be if you weren't pregnant, probably because pregnant women are very careful about avoiding injury. You are probably much more safety conscious now than ever before. Plus, you are more likely to be wearing flat shoes, choosing less-risky activities, and warming up and cooling down—all precautions that help you prevent injury.

However, if you do twist your ankle coming down the stairs or bump into your kitchen counter, your body is more likely to develop swelling and bruising. These minor inconveniences usually heal quickly.

What you really want to watch out for is injuring your belly. During your first trimester, your uterus is well protected behind the pubic bone. But as it grows higher into your belly, it is more likely to get injured because it sticks out. Plus, abrupt movements can cause problems inside your uterus. Avoid activities that put you at risk for injury to your belly, such as contact sports, ball sports, or ice sports. You can also modify your favorite activities to make them safer. If you love basketball, try competitive shooting rather than a contact game. If you are an experienced tennis player, try playing doubles rather than singles in order to reduce the strain on your joints. If you love winter sports, try cross-country skiing rather than downhill to avoid bad falls.

How will anemia affect my activities?

Few women develop anemia during pregnancy. If your doctor does diagnose you with anemia, it means that your iron levels are very low. This means your body cannot produce the red blood cells which deliver oxygen to your muscles and your fetus. So, you feel tired and worn out more quickly with exercise. Taking iron corrects this problem.

All pregnant women have slightly lower iron levels during pregnancy and this is normal—it's called "relative" anemia. This happens because our total blood volume increases during pregnancy, reducing the concentration of red blood cells, which carry iron. Throughout pregnancy, our bodies respond by producing more red blood cells—this is why you need extra iron, which you get in your prenatal vitamins. Even with this "relative" anemia, you can exercise because your body still gets all the oxygen it needs.

Does exercise stress the fetus?

Well, maybe a little—and that may be a good thing. When you work out regularly or warm up before exercising, you are conditioning your body to have more strength and stamina. You are probably also conditioning your fetus at the same time. This "training" may make your baby better able to deal with other stresses during gestation, such as a difficult labor. According to an article on exercise and fetal health in the *Journal of Developmental Physiology*, babies of active women show fewer signs of stress from not receiving enough oxygen or nutrients during labor and delivery. These babies are less likely to have a bowel movement in the amniotic fluid before birth (called *meconium*, which is potentially dangerous to the newborn) and more likely to have higher Apgar scores, a sign that they are well-adjusted and responsive at birth.

Will exercise reduce blood flow to my fetus?

It can—but only if you don't warm up before exercising or if you lie on your back after the first trimester. If you don't warm up gradually, your blood rushes to your skin and muscles—and away from your uterus—as soon as you start exercising. This can cause a temporary dip in your fetus's heart rate (called *bradycardia*). Don't worry: this brief dip is harmless and has no effect on your pregnancy. According to research presented in the journal *American Family Physician*, your fetus's heart rate returns to normal within a of couple minutes, with no negative effects.

The blood flow to the uterus may drop somewhat if you lie on your back after your first trimester. If you are sleeping, stretching, or doing floor exercises (like abdominal crunches) lying on your back, the whole weight of your uterus lies on top of your major blood vessels. This means that less blood reaches your heart and it cannot pump as efficiently. You may find that you feel dizzy or faint when you lie on your back—this is the reason. It is a lot healthier to lie on your side so that you do not obstruct your blood flow. All the stretches and exercises in this book will allow you to safely warm up and cool down without lying on your back for more than a few seconds.

Can exercise cause low blood sugar for me—and my fetus?

Yes, exercise uses up your blood sugar—but regular exercise may help you maintain healthier sugar level in the long run. If you exercise when you are very hungry, your blood sugar level may become too low. When you exercise, you burn fats and carbohydrates about six times faster than you do at rest. The carbohydrates you eat, such as starches and sugars, supply glucose—a sugar—to your muscles for immediate energy. With exercise, your blood sugar drops as your muscles use up the immediate supply of glucose in your blood. Low blood sugar may make you feel weak, ill, or headachy. These feelings are the body's signals to rest, eat, and drink. Your fetus depends on you for its nutrition, but as long as you have an adequately balanced diet overall, a brief period of low blood sugar (called *hypoglycemia*) will not harm your fetus.

When I exercise, does my fetus get enough oxygen?

Yes—your body almost guarantees it. Your body is extremely well adapted to do its job of maintaining a healthy supply of oxygen for your fetus, with increased blood volume, more efficient heart, and dilated blood vessels in the placenta and uterus. Plus, your fetus has a powerful ability to efficiently pick up oxygen from the blood—even if your oxygen level is low. This means that when you get out there and exercise, even if you feel short of breath, your fetus gets enough oxygen. What you should watch out for is exercising suddenly and strenuously, especially if you are not in good shape. Avoid sprinting after the mail truck or heading uphill right after snapping on your skis or hopping onto your bike. Take time to warm up, so that your body can always maintain a healthy blood flow to your fetus.

Is overheating dangerous for the fetus?

Yes—but getting a good workout and overheating are not the same thing. Heating up during exercise is healthy. Doing it in a hot tub or sauna is not healthy. Sweating, a result of a good workout, means your body's doing a little preventive cooling. Feeling dizzy, fatigued, flushed, and not sweating, whether from exercise or from the extreme heat of a hot tub or sauna, is a sign that you're too hot and dehydrated. If you get too hot, your fetus can also get too hot. This can affect its development, especially during the first trimester, when its organs are forming. Pregnancy is not the time to really push yourself, since if you overdo it, you can cause your body temperature to rise a couple degrees—and this may be enough to affect your fetus.

You're not likely to overheat while exercising. Most likely, you'll instinctively slow down and drink cool water as your body temperature rises. The longer and harder you exercise, or the warmer the weather, the more important it is that you stay cool, by removing layers of clothing, staying in the shade, and, most important, sweating.

Early in pregnancy, you'll notice that you become hot quickly. Overheating is less of a concern later in pregnancy. According to studies done by researcher R. W. Hale of elite athletes during pregnancy, women are better able to stay cool during the second and third trimesters. Later in pregnancy, your blood volume increases, you sweat more, and you have more blood sent to your skin, where it can cool off.

How can dehydration affect my pregnancy?

Listen up! Dehydration, which can happen quickly, is the one thing you really need to keep an eye on when exercising. If you have chapped lips, dry skin, a sticky mouth, or haven't urinated in over four hours, you may be dehydrated. If you become dehydrated, you are more susceptible to overheating, altitude illness, cold and heat illness, urinary infections, and even preterm labor.

To prevent dehydration, drink at least a liter of water per hour of exercise, and more if it is hot or humid. Drinking sports drinks or rehydration drinks that contain some salts will also help you stay better hydrated. If you've been vomiting, have diarrhea, or have a fever, you need extra fluids. Make a habit of maintaining good hydration during pregnancy—have a water bottle on hand whether you're at your desk, in the car, or heading out on the trail. Just having it with you will remind you to drink, whether you're thirsty or not.

Can I travel to higher altitudes during pregnancy?

If you live near sea level and have a healthy pregnancy, according to the American College of Obstetrics and Gynecology a short trip to moderate altitude—around six to eight thousand feet—should be safe for you and your fetus. This means flying is no problem, since commercial airplanes are pressurized at this altitude. Even some of the highest summits at ski resorts don't present a danger, especially since you probably won't be spending more than a few minutes at the top of the mountain anyway. So unless you're planning a high-altitude trek or heading out in an unpressurized plane (and I don't recommend either during pregnancy), you won't have to worry about altitude.

You've got to be careful about going above ten thousand feet, however. Dr. Peter Hackett, an altitude medicine expert, reviewed studies of women who live at sea level and spend time over ten thousand feet during pregnancy and showed

How to Prevent Problems at High Altitude During Pregnancy

- Exercise below six thousand feet (1,800 meters), especially if you live near sea level.

- Do not go above eight thousand feet (2,500 meters) in the first five days of altitude exposure. Then limit your exposure to altitudes of more than eight thousand feet to less than two hours (especially if you live at sea level).

- Do not go above ten thousand feet (3,000 meters) during pregnancy (especially if you live at sea level).

- Take time to get used to the altitude and descend at any signs of altitude illness, such as headache, nausea, vomiting, or shortness of breath. If you have trouble breathing at rest, difficulty walking, a cough with frothy pink sputum, or confusion, descend immediately and get medical attention.

- If you exercise within the first day or two of altitude exposure, start at the lowest possible altitude (not at the top of the mountain); the higher the altitude, the less strenuous your exercise should be.

- Take extra care to avoid dehydration and strenuous exercise at high altitude, since these (as well as alcohol and drugs) can worsen altitude illness.

- Women with any pregnancy-related problems should avoid any unnecessary altitude exposure.

- Avoid altitude exposure if you have habitually smoked more than half a pack a day in the last five years.

- Discuss any high-altitude travel plans with your doctor well before the trip.

that they can develop pregnancy complications. Of course, plenty of women live and give birth at high altitude, but their bodies are already adjusted. For someone from a lower elevation, it is likely that the combination of pregnancy, low oxygen levels, and exertion may dangerously affect the mother's and the fetus's endurance.

Can exercise cause premature labor?

No, no, and no! The common and unfortunate myth that exercise causes women to deliver prematurely keeps many healthy women indoors and sedentary. It is simply not true. Exercise can cause some irregular (sometimes sharp) contrac-

Red Flags to Watch Out for While Exercising

- Back or pelvic discomfort

- Belly pain

- Chest pain

- Contractions or tightening across your belly

- Decreased fetal movement

- Dizziness

- Headache

- Light-headedness

- Muscle weakness

- Nausea or vomiting

- Shortness of breath or feeling like you can't catch your breath

- Vaginal spotting or bleeding

tions, but these resolve after a few minutes of resting. In your late second and third trimesters, you may occasionally feel tightening across your belly with exercise; these are Braxton Hicks contractions, which do not lead to preterm labor. If you feel contractions, take a break, but don't stop exercising altogether. Studies reviewed in the journal *Birth* have shown that regular exercise may even protect against preterm labor, making it more likely for you to deliver safely at term.

This is an exciting time to be pregnant. Recent research has thrown out many of the myths that may have kept our mothers and grandmothers inactive during pregnancy. Exercise during pregnancy makes you stronger, more flexible, more energetic, and better prepared for the upcoming tasks of birthing and being a mother. It also promotes better fetal health and helps condition your fetus for the marathon of its own birth.

Medical Emergencies

Maybe fear of what could happen—that dreaded *emergency*—is keeping you from staying active during pregnancy. Well, it shouldn't. Of course, everyone defines an emergency differently. For you, an "emergency" may come to mean having an excruciatingly full bladder while stuck in a canoe in the middle of a lake. But in this section I want to alert you to the possible *medical* emergencies: injury to your belly, bleeding, contractions, and (yes, it could happen) going into labor.

The best thing you can do to prevent serious problems is to be aware of what symptoms to watch out for. These are your red flags. These symptoms let you know that you need to slow down and pay attention to your body.

Simple Steps You Can Take to Avoid an Emergency

- Tell someone responsible where you are going and when you will return.

- Talk about your plans with your doctor, especially if you have had any pregnancy complications.

- Exercise with someone responsible and capable at your side at all times.

- Carry a cell phone and make sure you stay in range.

- Carry a map of the area (including trails) and make note of ranger's stations and emergency phones.

- Wear comfortable gear that fits well and is safe for use in pregnancy.

- Always carry your doctor's office and after-hours phone numbers with you.

- Carry emergency phone numbers: someone with a car and keys to your house who is on call to pick you up and bring you to the hospital if necessary; someone who will call your work to make arrangements for your possible absence.

- Be aware of the shortest route to your car and the hospital (ideally reachable within thirty minutes).

- Near your due date, keep your hospital kit (the bag with everything you'll need in the hospital) in your car in case you go into labor.

- If you feel unwell or develop any disturbing symptoms, stop and rest immediately.

- Do not hesitate to get help.

Most likely, if you experience any worrisome symptoms you'll take a break, empty your bladder, drink some water, cool off, feel your baby kick, and be on your way. But just not feeling quite right is a good enough reason to call off your excursion and head back to the couch.

In a healthy pregnancy—if you take sensible precautions—moderate exercise outdoors will not cause complications. But, emergencies can arise any time. If something unexpected does happen, good preparation can prevent a setback from turning into an emergency.

Preventing Injury to Your Pregnant Belly

- Avoid situations where your belly is likely to be injured, such as contact sports, rough trails, ice or roller sports, and steep slopes—especially later in pregnancy.

- On a narrow trail or when walking in the dark, stay behind someone who can warn you of upcoming hazards.

- Wear your fanny pack, backpack straps, or seatbelt lap belt low across your hip bones, not across your belly.

- Head out only when you are comfortable with your equipment (such as a canoe or mountain bike) and know how to turn, slow down, and stop.

- On slippery surfaces or on a boat, stay low, hold on, and stay seated, if possible.

- Stick with a buddy who will be cautious, respect your limits, and look out for you.

- Get medical attention immediately if you are injured, fall, or are in any sort of accident.

Injury to the Pregnant Belly

Let's cut to the chase here and talk about preventing trauma. Got your flat shoes on? Holding the handrail when going down the stairs? Looking both ways a few times before crossing the parking lot? You've got it. As soon as you feel that belly poking out, you become protective of it—and that is a healthy instinct. You may have been comfortable taking some risks before pregnancy and not thinking too long and hard about potential injuries, but carrying a fetus should change all that. According to the *Journal of Trauma*, injury is the number one nonobstetric cause of maternal death and injury is the top cause of death in adults under age forty-five.

As you'd expect, the pregnant belly is pretty vulnerable to injury. By late pregnancy, it sticks out, pulls the body off balance, and allows the fetus to be tossed around with sudden movements or squished with direct pressure on the belly. In fact, the American College of Obstetrics and Gynecology reports that about one in twelve women will experience some trauma, however minor, during pregnancy.

Look Out for Signs of Labor

- Lightening (the feeling that your baby has dropped lower into your pelvis).

- Regular, strong contractions every five to six minutes (like menstrual cramps, a tightening across your belly, or a backache).

- Leaking fluid from the vagina, which would mean that your bag of water has broken.

- Passing bloody mucus from your vagina (your mucous plug or "bloody show").

But the fetus is also pretty well protected. During the first trimester, the uterus, with the developing fetus within, is shielded under the pubic bone. The fetus is also cushioned inside the thick-walled, muscular uterus and surrounded by amniotic fluid. As the pregnancy develops, however, the uterus grows into the belly and, by late pregnancy, pushes right up against the skin. This is when you can feel the baby kick just by putting your hand on your belly.

Keep in mind that you do not have to get slammed right on the belly to affect the pregnancy. Coming to a sudden stop (during a car accident or a fall onto your behind, for example) can cause a deceleration injury, meaning your uterus and placenta can get bent out of shape. And these injuries are *far* more common than any direct injury to the fetus itself. That's why getting help if you're in an accident is important, even if you don't think you hurt your belly and you feel just fine. You need to make sure your uterus, placenta, and fetus are fine too.

Bleeding

It doesn't take a lot of blood—a red streak on toilet paper will do it—to make you scream, "Emergency!" Yes, you'll need to get some medical help, but don't panic yet. Minor bleeding, or spotting, is a common symptom during pregnancy, especially during your first trimester. Being active or having sex will not cause significant bleeding. But bleeding can signify a problem and only a doctor's exam (and maybe an ultrasound to look directly at the fetus) can ultimately reassure you.

Vaginal bleeding during pregnancy has many different causes—some much less worrisome than others. One common cause of early-pregnancy bleeding is menstruating a little as your body adjusts to pregnancy hormonal levels.

However, bleeding may signify more serious problems. Bleeding is a symptom of miscarriage, which occurs in 15 to 20 percent of pregnancies in healthy, fertile women, and often cannot be prevented. Bleeding may be a sign of an ectopic pregnancy (a relatively rare condition in which the pregnancy is inside the fallopian tube), which can require immediate surgery.

In later pregnancy, infection, cervical changes, or a low placenta can cause a little spotting. If you're bleeding, your doctor will want to check that your placenta and uterus are not at risk. And you'll want to make sure you're not going into labor (remember, it starts with a "bloody show"). If you see red at any point during your pregnancy, get help.

Contractions

It is one of the most frequent concerns about exercise that women voice: *what about the contractions?* It's true: in late pregnancy, rigorous exercise often triggers contractions. But it's not necessarily an emergency. The contractions typically go away if you just rest for a few minutes.

Contractions are the sensation of the muscular uterus readying itself to birth the fetus. They may feel like a tightening across the abdomen or an ache in the lower back. Unlike other pain, labor contractions come and go in intervals, becoming stronger, more regular, and more frequent. With exercise, you may feel Braxton Hicks contractions. You can distinguish them from real labor by the fact that they are irregular; they do not get closer together; they stop when you change position or rest; they may be uncomfortable but do not become increasingly painful; and they are generally only felt across your belly, not in your back.

During exercise, you may develop contractions for several reasons: dehydration, strenuous exercise, injury—or simply being near your due date.

If you are at term—within three weeks of your due date—you should head to the hospital (to the labor and delivery area) if you are having regular contractions approximately every five minutes or are leaking fluid. If you are more than three weeks from your due date and have contractions that don't go away in a few minutes, you should see your doctor to be evaluated for preterm labor.

What to Do if You Feel Contractions While Exercising

- Stop exercising and take a break.

- If you can, lie down on your left side while you wait for the contractions to stop.

- Check for other signs of labor, such as leaking fluid (if you have broken your bag of water) or bloody mucus (called the "bloody show").

- Time the contractions. If they continue at regular intervals and become stronger, you are in labor: call your doctor and get to a hospital.

- If the contractions stop within a few minutes, continue to exercise cautiously and take frequent breaks to hydrate, catch your breath, and feel for more contractions.

Going into Labor

As much as we'd like to be able to predict and plan around our delivery date, the truth is that we never know when we're going to go into labor. Remember that, on average, half of all women deliver in the three weeks *before* their due date. Many doctors encourage light exercise for women who are near term or past their due date. Exercising outdoors may help you burn off that last-minute nervous anticipation, pass the time near your due date, stay relaxed, and even help get those contractions going more regularly.

No matter how far along you are in your pregnancy, you have already learned that pregnancy is full of surprises, not all of them pleasant. Knowing what to watch out for and what to worry about is key to keeping your cool and protecting yourself.

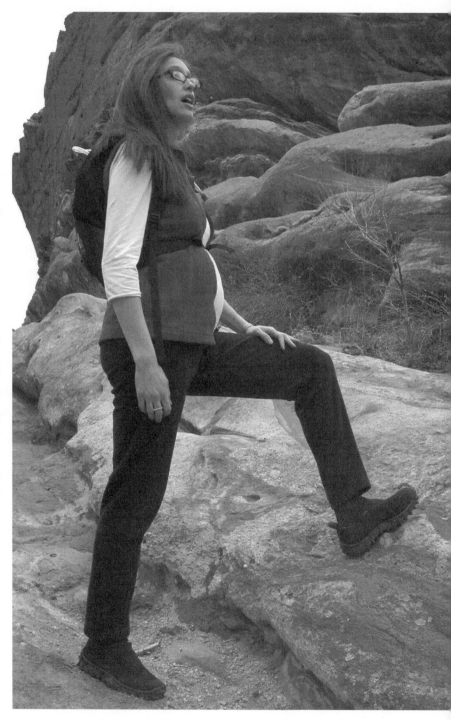

Staying Healthy
Each Trimester

During pregnancy, your body will go through amazing changes, even more drastic and awe-inspiring than those of adolescence. Your pregnancy will also change how you view your future, your relationships, and your body. Within a few days—or hours—of that positive pregnancy test, you'll realize that you are fundamentally responsible for the fetus growing inside you and should start treating your body with special care.

Exercise can help you cope with some of the immediate changes during pregnancy and help alleviate some aches and pains. On the other hand, some of the symptoms you may experience each trimester will certainly affect how you exercise. As any mother will tell you, each trimester presents its own challenges and rewards when it comes to staying active. To get the most out of your activities while protecting yourself and your fetus, develop a good relationship with your doctor and seek his or her advice.

Involve Your Doctor

Have you talked with your doctor about your outdoor activities? No? Then you're like most women who don't mention the diverse ways they stay active during pregnancy. And your doctor probably won't ask. But if you stay silent, you may

Pregnancy Complications that May Interfere with Exercise

- Pregnancy-induced hypertension (high blood pressure caused by pregnancy)

- Premature labor

- Uterine or vaginal bleeding

- Incompetent cervix (cervix that starts dilating too early)

- Premature rupture of membranes (broken bag of water)

- Placenta previa (placenta covering the cervix) in the third trimester

- A history of preterm deliveries

be passing up a terrific opportunity to learn a lot more about your body and get some solid advice about what is safe for you and your fetus.

The word *exercise* means different things to different people. Have you been exercising? Well, maybe you did spend a half hour on a treadmill or at a prenatal swim class. More than likely, you have been doing lots of other kinds of exercise too, like raking leaves on a Saturday afternoon or biking to work. Our definition of *exercise* is broader than in the past. During pregnancy, everything you do to stay active counts. You don't have to stick with a prescribed routine to make an activity worthwhile. Walking one day and kayaking the next is all good exercise. Go ahead and mention your activities to your doctor.

Your obstetrician will be interested in how often and how rigorously you exercise so that she can develop a good sense of your level of fitness. Revisit the topic during your monthly visits as your exercise regimen evolves with your pregnancy and the changing weather. As you plan an upcoming vacation, discuss the activities you are looking forward to, especially if you haven't tried them yet during pregnancy. Also, talk about how you will be getting there and where you will be staying. Your doctor can offer valuable advice on health issues such as preventing blood clots during long car rides and acclimatizing when you go to a higher altitude.

If your doctor expresses concern about a certain activity, make sure you understand why. There may be some risks you and your doctor agree on, but some where your doctor may err on the side of caution. For example, some outdoor activities are considerably safer if you are experienced but can be risky for novices. In addition, things like slightly elevated blood pressure, the location of the placenta over your cervix, a heart murmur, or the fetus's health may affect your doctor's comfort with your exercising—especially if you are heading into the wilderness or are training rigorously.

On the other hand, you may think you can't exercise in certain situations—such as near your due date or if you have diabetes, insomnia, ankle swelling, back soreness, or mood swings—when your doctor would recommend that you can and should. You can be sure you are maximizing your exercise regimen if you discuss it with your doctor first.

First Trimester: Your First Three Months

The first few months of your pregnancy are the most extraordinary and over-whelming—even though no one can see that you are pregnant yet. Your preg-nancy will certainly make itself obvious to you however. The early changes of pregnancy can be hard to cope with because you can feel so different—and, frankly, unwell—most of the time. You may not feel energetic or motivated enough to exercise because your body is devoting all of its energy to your devel-oping fetus. It's okay to be lazy and pamper yourself a little. But keep in mind that exercise can help you stay relaxed, gain confidence in your rapidly changing body, and make you feel better.

Within weeks, you will develop some telltale signs of pregnancy that affect how you feel—and how you exercise. For one thing, you will notice that your breasts grow significantly in the first two months, especially if you are small chested. Your breasts will feel tender and sensitive and the bouncing and friction during activity—like running or skiing—may be quite uncomfortable. Look for firmly supportive sports bras that fit well so your breasts don't become more ten-der with exercise. Demi bras, underwires, and lace and synthetic fabrics may be particularly irritating. If your nipples are especially sensitive, you may want to protect them with cloth nursing pads when you are active.

Another common symptom that women notice early in pregnancy is hav-ing to urinate more often. As your uterus grows, it puts pressure on your blad-der, making you feel like you really have to go. The sensation improves during your second trimester but becomes much more obvious again during your third trimester, when the baby rests on your bladder. It may feel like you just got out on the trail and have to stop for another "call of nature." This is normal—just

Good Activities for Your First Trimester

- Biking

- In-line skating

- Running

- Skiing and snowboarding

- Snorkeling

- Surfing

- Windsurfing

take it in stride. Take lots of breaks and choose activities with places where you can urinate: it just won't be as much fun if you've got a bursting bladder. And despite your frequent need to urinate, keep drinking a lot of fluids, especially if you are active, to avoid dehydration.

You may also notice that you develop varicose veins: on your legs, around your breasts, on your belly, on your vulva—even around your anus, called hemorrhoids—during the first trimester. These visible and sometimes painful surface veins are normal during pregnancy because your body is suddenly circulating so much more blood. Most varicose veins resolve gradually after delivery, but regular, gentle exercise, like swimming, cross-country skiing, and walking, can help prevent minor varicose veins from forming or getting worse. Also, elevating your legs after exercising will help prevent blood from pooling in your legs and making varicose veins more obvious. If you have to stand or sit for long periods, take breaks to walk and stretch and try wearing support stockings to improve your circulation and minimize varicose veins.

Since your hormones fluctuate wildly in the first couple of months of pregnancy, you also experience a host of other symptoms that can make you feel lousy, like nausea, cramping, fatigue, insomnia, irritability, and depression. Getting outside, exercising, and taking good care of yourself will help you get through this tough period, improving your mood, appetite, and sleep patterns.

If you're worried about protecting your fetus, know the first trimester is a very good time for you to enjoy outdoor activities, since your uterus is safely tucked behind your pubic bone, protected in case you fall or are hit in the belly. If you feel up to it, go ahead and learn to cross-country ski or start swimming. Most of the activities discussed in this book are pretty safe during your first trimester—particularly if you've done them before and you use a good dose of common sense. Your main concerns should be keeping hydrated, taking frequent breaks, and staying cool. Remember that your fetus's organs are developing at this time and elevated body temperature can be dangerous. But this shouldn't stop you from exercising regularly and breaking a sweat.

Listen to your body. If you don't feel like exercising during the first few months of pregnancy, fine. But if your pregnancy is healthy overall, remember that some regular activity now will make you feel healthier throughout your pregnancy—and afterward. During your second trimester, your body will start to work in harmony and you'll feel better overall—and you may feel more motivated to stay active.

Second Trimester: Your Fourth Through Sixth Months

During your second trimester, you'll experience one of the biggest rewards of pregnancy—feeling your baby's movement. Some women say that this exciting sensation, called *quickening*, is like feeling a tiny dolphin swimming inside you. Soon you'll be able to associate the movements with actual body parts pressed against the front of your growing belly: a head, a back, a foot. This is when you really start bonding with your baby, and you may even notice that he or she responds differently when you exercise. At this point in pregnancy, your fetus can hear music and certainly feels the rhythm of your movements.

Many women feel increased energy and comfort with their bodies during their second trimester—the body has reached a kind of equilibrium. You are also done with some of the most uncomfortable sensations of pregnancy: the nausea and fatigue. However, the second trimester comes with some unique symptoms that may affect your exercise routine.

A common symptom during the second (and third) trimester is pelvic pain. This sharp and often sudden pain is caused by your rapidly growing uterus stretching your round ligaments, which suspend the uterus in the pelvis. For many women, this pain becomes worse with walking and running. You may find that one side aches more than the other; this is normal. Resting regularly and doing some dynamic stretching (see chapter 6) may help alleviate this pain.

Another common complaint during the second trimester is back pain—and it can also get a lot better with regular stretching and exercise. Your back aches because your growing belly changes your center of gravity, causing your back to arch and putting a lot of strain on your lower back muscles, which are just getting used to holding up your heavier body. Wear comfortable, supportive

Good Activities for Your Second Trimester

- **Cross-country skiing**
- **Hiking**
- **Paddling**
- **Sailing**
- **Snorkeling**
- **Swimming**

shoes to keep your back in line—high heels will cause you to arch your back more severely. Also, wear a very supportive bra, especially if you have large breasts, because you may also experience some upper back pain as your breasts continue to grow and become heavier.

Your uterus has grown well out of your pelvis and your belly has started to stick out. This means that your fetus is more vulnerable to injury, so you have to start being careful about avoiding falls and activities where you could get forcefully bumped. This is not the time to play pickup basketball or learn to in-line skate. Check the risk assessment for each activity in this book to rule out riskier outdoor activities, like downhill skiing, snowboarding, windsurfing, and mountain biking.

Now that your uterus is much larger, you may feel dizzy if you lie on your back. In this position, the uterus puts pressure on your major blood vessels, reducing the blood flow back to your heart and to the rest of your body—including your fetus. Accordingly, choose exercises and stretches where you are upright or on your side.

Other common complaints during the second trimester—and continuing through delivery—are constipation and bloating. Regular, moderate exercise can help relieve these problems because it gets your bowels moving—as long as you also keep yourself well hydrated and eat plenty of fiber in fruits, cereals, and wheat bread.

You may also start to experience some ankle swelling and water retention during the second trimester. Gentle exercise can help improve your circulation and reduce swelling, although the best remedy is to elevate your feet after activity and avoid standing still for long periods.

Although you may notice that you don't have to go to the bathroom as frequently during your second trimester (your uterus has lifted so it is above your bladder temporarily), you may occasionally leak some urine, especially when you cough or sneeze. This loss of bladder control is caused by the stretching of the pelvic floor muscles in preparation for delivery. Exercise helps tone the muscles to prevent leakage—specifically Kegel exercises focus on strengthening your pelvic muscles. If you are heading out of the house, especially after your twentieth week, wear a pad in your underwear, just in case—but don't worry, these muscles will gradually tighten up again after delivery.

Your second trimester is a great time to get in shape, taking advantage of your increasing comfort with your pregnant body and your increasing energy. If you establish a regular exercise regimen this trimester—even if you didn't exercise during the first few months of pregnancy—you will enjoy the benefits from now through delivery. Plus, exercise is a special way to bond with your growing baby, since he can feel your movements and you can feel his.

Third Trimester: Your Seventh Month Through Delivery

Your third trimester is a time of preparation and, hopefully, patience. You and your partner will be getting your lives in order to accommodate your new family member and preparing psychologically for one of the biggest transitions of your life. Chances are that well before your due date, you'll feel ready to give birth and start this phase of your life. This is where the patience comes in. You may be feeling so big that everything takes twice as long and you can't imagine moving around too much at all. Meanwhile, your fetus is gaining weight and doing a lot of aerobic activity—you'll feel those kicks and somersaults day and night.

The more you managed to exercise earlier in pregnancy, the more active you'll be during your third trimester. Any regular exercise will pay off with more stamina, strength, and flexibility. You'll be enjoying less back and pelvic pain, less shortness of breath, and less trouble moving around. I'm not saying you won't have those problems—you will simply be better off and more likely to get out and about during this trimester.

When you get the results of your glucose screening test, a blood test routinely done around twenty-four to twenty-eight weeks, you may also discover that you have borderline high blood sugar or outright gestational diabetes (problems controlling your sugar level during pregnancy). Regular exercise can help control your blood sugar—both preventing and helping to treat diabetes.

Good Activities for Your Third Trimester

- **Canoeing**
- **Dynamic stretching**
- **Gardening**
- **Snowshoeing**
- **Swimming**
- **Walking**

One of the most common complaints during the third trimester is back pain. Obviously, you are carrying the growing fetus, amniotic fluid, a large uterus, and all the extra blood and muscles needed to support the pregnancy. You probably weigh about twenty-five pounds more than you did a year ago. And your fetus is gaining about seven ounces per week.

This extra weight causes a drastic shift in your center of gravity, shifting it forward and putting great strain on your lower back. You'll need to consciously work on your posture to keep your back straight, whether you are stretching, exercising, lifting your toddler or a bag of groceries, or sitting at your desk. If you have upper back pain too, wear a supportive bra, hold your shoulders back, and lift your chest so that your growing breasts don't strain your shoulder and back muscles.

At around thirty-two weeks, the aches and pains in your hips and pelvis will peak as the pelvic joints and ligaments relax in preparation for delivery. Because of the tenderness in your pelvis and around your uterus in general—many women feel pain right under the ribs—high-impact sports (those with a lot of bouncing, like running) are not a good choice. Many women find that they get really sore tailbones because the sacroiliac joint at the bottom of the back bears the weight of the pregnancy. Sitting for long periods, especially on hard surfaces, may be very uncomfortable. This may be something to consider if you are going sailing or boating and will be sitting on a wooden seat or deck—bring extra cushions, lean against something, and get up and walk around whenever you can.

As the pregnancy progresses and the baby wedges her head into the pelvis, you'll feel even more pressure in the pelvis. Plus, you'll notice that the baby is sitting right on top of your bladder again, so you will want to pick activities that allow you to use the bathroom frequently. For example, kayaking and cross-country skiing may become very inconvenient, but gardening and walking near home may seem much more attractive.

It is also normal to retain some fluid at this point in pregnancy and you may see your feet, ankles, lower legs, and even hands and wrists swell up. This can make it harder to simply get into your shoes, but it can also lead to some stiffness and pain that may interfere with your movement. The swelling sometimes causes a harmless burning and itching on the soles of your feet; sitting down and putting your feet up will help relieve the discomfort. Exercising in the mornings, when the swelling is less pronounced, will help you stay in shape and will improve your circulation during the rest of the day.

Because this swelling puts pressure on nerves in your wrist, carpal tunnel syndrome is more common late in pregnancy. If you develop carpal tunnel syndrome, you'll feel tingling in your index, middle, and ring fingers. Don't worry: it will resolve after delivery. Wearing a splint at night may help. If you develop carpal tunnel symptoms, stay away from activities that strain your wrists, like paddling or cross-country skiing.

The minute you get up to do something active during your third trimester, you'll notice one thing: you are huffing and puffing. This is because your baby is taking up all the space in your belly and is pressing up against your diaphragm, making it difficult for you to get a deep breath. It doesn't mean that you are out of shape or that your baby is short of oxygen—it just means that you may have to wait for her to change position. Closer to your due date, your baby will settle down into your pelvis and move away from your lungs, making it easier for you to breathe and get some exercise. As I've said before, the better shape you're in, the more efficiently your lungs will work to deliver oxygen and the less you will need those deep breaths when you do simple activities.

During the end of your second trimester and throughout your third, you will also notice some mini-contractions—especially when you exercise and raise your heart rate. These are called Braxton Hicks, or "false labor," contractions. Having these contractions, which can feel quite sharp, does not mean that you are going into labor. These are your body's dress rehearsal for labor, but they don't cause your cervix to open or your bag of water to break. It can be frightening to feel this tightening across your belly, especially if you are not close to your due date. But you can tell the difference between these and real labor. How? First of all, Braxton Hicks contractions will go away when you rest for a few minutes or change position. Real labor contractions will just get stronger and stronger. Secondly, these contractions are usually irregular and sudden, rather than the gradual and rhythmic contractions of real labor. Finally, you will feel Braxton Hicks contractions only across your belly, while real labor typically involves both your belly and back. Or you may never feel Braxton Hicks contractions at all—that's normal too.

Labor and Delivery

And then finally the show is on and your body wholeheartedly goes into labor. You will feel increasingly potent contractions and you'll know that your cervix is starting to open. Your doctor may encourage you to get up and walk around during early labor. Early labor contractions, which soften the cervix and prepare it for labor, may start days or even weeks before you deliver. Walking will help make your contractions more regular, help your cervix open more quickly, and let gravity do some of the work of bringing your baby down into your pelvis. Just keep breathing through those contractions and get to the hospital delivery room if your water breaks. Doing some stretches between contractions will help keep your back, shoulder, and neck muscles relaxed during labor and make you more comfortable, especially after you've been laboring in bed for a long time. When your contractions are coming five minutes apart, your doctor will tell you to come to the hospital.

If you kept up some regular cardiovascular exercise during your nine months, like swimming, raking leaves, jogging, or cross-country skiing, your heart and lungs will have terrific stamina for labor. Pushing your baby through the pelvis requires strong pelvic floor muscles. You tone those muscles (as well as many others) by exercising against resistance, such as biking, doing water aerobics, hiking uphill, and padding out on your board to catch some surf. Stretching consistently improves your flexibility, which you will rely on when pulling up your knees to push. Regular exercise also trains your body to release endorphins—those "feel good" chemicals that will flood your system during labor and cause you to feel less pain. Even if you have a Cesarean section, your level of fitness will speed your recovery, since toned muscles heal faster and exercisers recuperate more quickly from anesthesia and surgery. Enjoying a variety of activities is the best preparation for the triathlon of labor and delivery.

This is where you will reap many of the benefits of staying active during pregnancy: most likely, your labor will be easier, you'll feel less worn out and require less anesthesia, you'll have a smaller chance of complications, and you'll probably need fewer medical interventions. Now, doesn't that feel good?

Your body goes through fantastic changes during pregnancy and each trimester—really, each *day*—brings new surprises in the form of uncomfortable symptoms and the joyous emotions as your baby grows and flourishes inside you. Exercise is a healthy part of this process and can help you cope not only with the daily demands and stresses but also with the physical changes of pregnancy. Now that you are familiar with these common complaints—and how exercise affects them—you can design an exercise regimen you feel comfortable with. Pick activities you truly enjoy so that you'll stay motivated to be active throughout pregnancy and well after, when your baby can appreciate the outdoors with you.

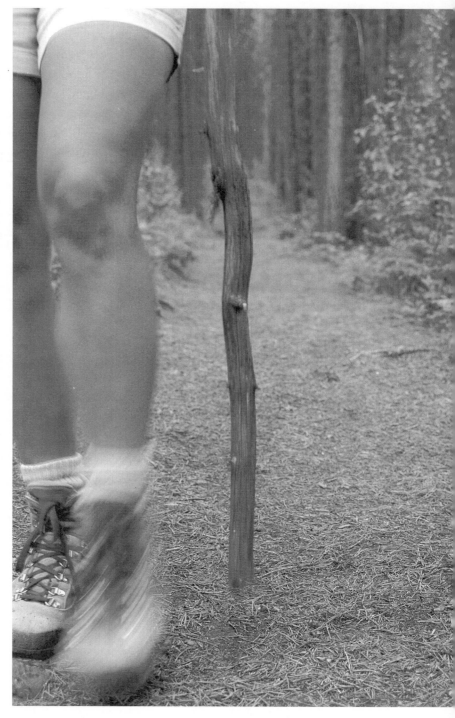

chapter 4

Outdoor Gear
for Pregnancy

You may have had no trouble buying maternity wear well before you needed it, but you'll have a harder time finding maternity outdoor gear even when you really need it. Fortunately, most of the outdoor equipment you already own will serve you well during pregnancy. However, there are a few factors that you may wish to consider, especially if you are in the market for new gear. Remember that choosing good gear is not just about comfort, although that may seem most important—it is about protecting yourself from heat and cold exposure, supporting your vulnerable joints, accommodating your expanding belly, preventing injury, and providing essential hydration and nutrition. That's a lot to ask of your equipment, so it pays to choose your gear carefully.

Exercise Clothing

You may have given up on making any fashion statements during your pregnancy, but when you exercise, what you wear matters. Choose clothing that offers you the best protection against sunburn, rain or snow, insect bites, falls, and overheating.

Wear layers. Close to the skin, wear breathable fabrics, such as silk, cotton, or synthetics designed for insulation and breathability, such as polypropylene-based Capilene or Thermastat. For warmer weather, or strenuous activities in the snow such as cross-country skiing, wear lightweight underwear. In cold weather, choose heavyweight undergarments that wick away moisture and keep you warm and dry. In general, wear layers so that you can maintain a comfortable temperature, since sweating too much can make you dehydrated and overheating can be dangerous.

Cover exposed skin. During pregnancy, you are more susceptible to sunburn and insect bites, so long sleeves and pants are best, even in warm temperatures. Also, these can protect you from minor bruises, scratches, and skin reactions to contact with wild plants. For most outdoor activities, your most comfortable maternity clothing will work well—elastic-waist pants or sweatpants to fit over your belly, a t-shirt, and a long-sleeved shirt, plus, in colder weather, a sweater and a large jacket that closes snugly around your belly.

Be prepared for weather changes. In cool weather, don't forget a hat, scarf, and gloves, since you may be more susceptible to hypothermia (or cold illness). For snow activities, wear water-resistant pants and jacket and tuck insulating undergarments into snow pants to minimize your cold and wetness exposure. Be prepared for sudden changes in weather with a packable lightweight rain and windproof jacket with a hood. For longer excursions into the wilderness, keep nighttime conditions in mind even if you are only planning a day trip, in case of an emergency.

Protect your breasts. With tender breasts, a sports bra can offer good support during activity. As breasts enlarge, underwire bras can become uncomfortable and your old bras may become too tight; during exercise, the bra rubbing against your tender nipples can cause abrasions. The solution is to find a well-fitting sports bra with good padding and applying petroleum jelly to the nipples to prevent abrasion.

Buy other specialty maternity clothing for your outdoor activities only if you find it more comfortable, such as maternity swimsuits, leggings, and jeans. The basic rule is that if you are comfortable, you have chosen the right clothing for the activity.

Footwear

During your pregnancy, your changing balance and shape affect your choices in footwear. Although convenient slip-ons may be your first choice in the house, sturdy and supportive footwear is key when you head outside, especially for exercise. Convenience is still important, though, since your growing belly may interfere with your being able to pull on or off boots or lace up shoes.

Your joints and ligaments relax during pregnancy. This adaptation, caused by the body's release of the hormone relaxin, allows the pelvis to expand to accommodate the baby's head as it passes through the narrow pelvic structure. However, the combination of relaxed joints and a change in a woman's center of gravity lead to an unsteady gait. One good way to prevent falls is to choose comfortable, appropriate footwear, and there are many varieties to choose from.

Footwear for Pregnancy: Buying Tips

- **Look for easy closure.** Footwear with Velcro or elastic closures is considerably easier to manage during pregnancy, especially once your belly prevents you from bending forward, crouching, or reaching your own shoes.

- **Shop later in the day.** Shopping for footwear after you have already been on your feet for several hours or after a hike is the best way to find out how well those shoes will fit when your feet become swollen after a few hours of exercise.

- **Get a good fit.** Before lacing up, put on the shoe or boot and slide your foot as far forward as it will go. If you can slip just one finger behind your heel, it should be a good fit. Then lace (or strap) up and stand up on the balls of your feet; if your heel slides up and down, this shoe may be too big and could cause blisters. Walk down a sharp incline if possible; if your toes jam the front of the shoe, you need a bigger size.

- **Try it with socks.** When buying shoes or boots, wear the same socks (and insoles) that you plan to wear while outdoors.

- **Break them in.** To avoid discomfort and blisters, take time to break in your shoes before heading out.

Running shoes are best for activities that involve primarily forward movement because they have a thick heel wedge, which tilts the body forward. A good running shoe for pregnancy may be a slightly larger size than you're used to. The running shoe should be lightweight and have a firm, shock-absorbent midsole and a breathable upper, to allow for sweating.

Walking and hiking shoes should absorb the shock of a paved or uneven surface. Good walking shoes have a rubber heel. Shoes designed for longer hikes may have curved soles to facilitate the rocking movement of walking. Walking and hiking footwear, whether you choose athletic-type shoes or boots, should provide firm support along both sides of your foot and under your arch, since your arch also relaxes during pregnancy. Boots offer better ankle support than shoes do, which is important if you are changing direction often or walking on an uneven surface. Choose a boot that has enough flexibility to accommodate your swollen feet without cutting off your circulation. Keep in mind that wearing heavy boots, such as those with steel siding, will increase your workout and your fatigue.

Cross-training shoes are a good choice if you enjoy a variety of activities and don't want to buy separate shoes for each. They work well for running, walking, and start-and-stop sports such as basketball or tennis. These are also a good choice for mountain biking and camping, since you need a shoe that is comfortable for wearing in camp, on the bike, and on the trail. You can also wear cross trainers comfortably on a boat or when paddling, since they offer good traction and the fabric uppers dry quickly. Cross trainers could become your favorite shoes during your first and second trimesters, since they offer good heel support (you'll need it as you gain weight), are breathable (for sweaty pregnant feet), and provide some ankle support (for those relaxed and sprain-prone ankles).

Athletic sandals are ideal for water sports since they are designed to get wet and dry quickly. While you may be used to wearing rubber-soled sandals with buckles or Velcro straps while paddling, fishing, or sailing, these sandals offer little arch or ankle support. They may be comfortable for wearing on the deck or in the kayak, since they allow your foot to breathe and are easily adjustable to your changing foot size, but they are not a good choice for walking. If you use sandals on a boat, choose a pair with excellent traction, a thick sole, and firm heel support.

44

Insoles are often recommended during pregnancy to improve the shock absorption of ordinary athletic shoes. However, your best option is to buy shoes that are designed for the activity you pursue most regularly, since a good shoe will offer good cushioning as well as support your arch and ankle. A good reason to use insoles is if they make your feet more comfortable either by supplementing the support of a worn sole or by providing better arch support. Some women find that standing for long periods during pregnancy is less taxing to their back and legs if they wear shoes with insoles. Certain types of insoles may cause your feet to overheat and, therefore, may increase the sweating and swelling in your feet. When choosing insoles, be sure to try them with the shoes you intend to put them in and try several types before deciding which works best for you.

Socks are another important aspect of footwear. Well-fitted socks that wick away moisture from your feet may help prevent abrasions and blisters and even control foot swelling caused by overheating. Maintain good circulation to your feet by making sure socks are pulled smoothly over your feet, with no wrinkles, especially in cold weather.

The placement of protective padding on various athletic socks varies—at the heel, ball, instep, arch, or shin. This padding can help support your foot and prevent rubbing that causes blisters (although the best prevention is a pair of shoes or boots that fit well). Choose your socks according to weather as well; use warm wool socks for snowshoeing or skiing and quick-drying socks for canoeing or biking. Since you sweat more during pregnancy, always choose socks that remove moisture from your feet. Thin nylon socks offer no support and they encourage blisters by keeping your skin moist.

Support stockings can help to alleviate the discomfort of varicose veins and ankle swelling during pregnancy. These stockings, which cover the shins or even the entire thighs, help to circulate the blood in the legs, which tends to pool in dilated veins during pregnancy. Your stockings should not bunch behind the knees, since this can impede circulation.

Exercise may help relieve ankle swelling by working your leg muscles and improving circulation. However, some women may experience swelling from spending more time on their feet while exercising. In this case, support stockings may help—and may even relieve the feeling of fatigue.

Bags and Packs

Carrying your water, food, and supplies with you—and keeping them accessible—can be a challenge during pregnancy. Toting bags increases your weight and exertion; can place uncomfortable pressure on your belly and breasts; puts strain on your back; and may even throw off your balance and lead to an injury.

When choosing and packing your bag or pack, consider both comfort and safety, and choose one that fits your pregnant body well. During pregnancy, you need to minimize the strain on your back. More important, you need to avoid pressure across your abdomen, which can affect your uterus. Although no studies have examined the effects of extended gentle pressure on the uterus—such as from backpack hip straps—the effects of pressure injury are well known from studies looking at safety belt trauma in car accidents. To protect your uterus when wearing a bag or pack, use the same precautions as you do for a seatbelt throughout pregnancy (see below), especially after the first trimester, when the fetus is no longer protected below the pubic bone.

How to Wear a Bag or Pack During Pregnancy

- The hip straps on a backpack can minimize the strain on your back and shoulders and should be placed *under* your pregnant belly, *not* across your belly.

- Hip straps for a backpack or fanny pack should cross over the bony crests of your pelvic bones on both sides and connect over the pubic bone, so the weight falls on these bones.

- In order to take the weight of the pack off your back, the hip straps should be pulled snugly, without slack, so that the weight rests on your hips.

- The backpack's structure should allow for some breathing space between the pack and your back to minimize contact sweating and allow ventilation.

- Any shoulder bags should be slung diagonally from one shoulder to the other hip, in order to distribute the weight. The strap should run between the breasts, rather than just over one shoulder or over one arm.

Whether you choose a backpack with an internal or external frame depends on your needs. An **internal frame backpack** is lighter and may therefore be easier to carry during pregnancy. Also, it does not have an awkward frame that can snag on branches and cause falls. However, an **external frame backpack** has advantages during pregnancy as well. It distributes weight more evenly, so you carry the weight higher up on your body and put less strain on the back and shoulders.

Sleeping Gear

There is essentially no sleeping gear made especially for pregnant women. If you plan to camp overnight in the wilderness, however, you will need to make sure your sleeping bag is warm enough and that your pad is comfortable. For some women, a hammock is also useful during pregnancy.

The most important rule for sleeping gear is that it must allow you to sleep comfortably on your side—preferably your left side. This is because after about twenty weeks' gestation, the weight of your uterus when you lie on your back or right side can obstruct the blood flow through your major vessels, affecting the fetus. Sleeping on your left side minimizes the pressure on the big vein that returns blood to your heart.

Sleeping bags. Since you will try to sleep on your left side during pregnancy, you will probably want a sleeping bag with a left-sided zipper. Most sleeping bags come with either a right or left opening—if you have one of each, the two bags can be zipped together to form a double bed. If you are buying a sleeping bag during pregnancy, choose one with a wide girth to allow for your pregnant belly. Not all sleeping bags are the same size. Most come in regular or long lengths, but different brands will have different widths. Also, remember your susceptibility to temperature changes during pregnancy: use a sleeping bag that is more than adequate for low nightly temperatures.

Hammocks. If you plan to sleep in a hammock, try it out beforehand to be sure you will be comfortable sleeping on your side. Choose a hammock with spreader bars at the ends to help keep the hammock flat. Hang it securely at a height that allows you to straddle the hammock with both your feet firmly on the ground when getting in and out.

Sleeping pads. During pregnancy, a good sleeping pad can help offer some back support and prevent soreness. Test foam and inflatable pads to determine which allow you to change position comfortably and insulate you well from the ground. Foam pads with a waterproof cover and convoluted foam offer better insulation and support than a simple flat foam pad. Some foam pads also convert to camp chairs—offering an excellent way to get off your feet, especially during pregnancy.

Life Jackets

During pregnancy, you may be at greater risk of drowning because of impaired balance and decreased lung capacity. Wearing a life jacket, or personal flotation device (PFD), on the water is very important and is required by law in some states. Any life jacket you wear should be Coast Guard–approved. If you need to rent or buy a life jacket, pick one that is appropriate for the conditions. A Type I PFD is the best for all conditions and will turn you faceup if you become unconscious. A Type II PFD is safe on inland, calm waters and may be more comfortable during pregnancy. A Type III PFD is safe only if you are a strong swimmer and are in shallow water—do not use this jacket for water sports, such as windsurfing or kayaking.

Check the label of the life jacket for size and weight limitations (the life jacket you wore before pregnancy will probably not fit you during your third trimester). A life jacket fits well if the straps and buckles fit securely around your belly and the jacket does not bunch up around your chest or slip back over your head.

Snacks and Drinks

Keeping yourself well fed and hydrated is essential for your pregnancy and, especially outdoors, for preventing serious problems such as heat exhaustion, cold illness, and altitude sickness, which are all more likely to occur if you are dehydrated. Drinking plenty of water and eating regular snacks can also help prevent nausea and motion sickness.

Food. During pregnancy, your body requires 300 additional calories per day. Especially when you exercise, it is important to maintain an adequate diet and healthy weight gain. While exercising, keep snacks available and eat small meals throughout the day. Healthy, portable options include nuts, fruit, crackers, dried fruit, gorp ("good old raisins and peanuts"), and granola bars. Sugary sweets, such as candy bars, provide less long-term energy, but they can be included in a balanced diet. Keep your snacks in a buddy's backpack or in your fanny pack, where you can reach them easily.

Water. You need to drink a liter of water per hour of exercise. If it is hot or humid or you are really exerting yourself, you may need more. The best solution for easy access to water is to carry a hydration pack on your back with a flexible straw you can sip from. These packs are lightweight, are comfortable to wear even during pregnancy, and will encourage you to stay hydrated.

If you become severely dehydrated, sports hydration drinks can help replace your salts (electrolytes). Caffeinated beverages such as soda, tea, or coffee do not provide good hydration; instead, they cause the body to lose water.

Packing Checklist

Make sure you are carrying all the essentials for a safe day outdoors. What you need will depend on the terrain, the weather, and your planned excursion. During pregnancy, it is especially important for you to be prepared for weather changes, carry more than sufficient water and food, and be able to get help quickly if you need it. See the Outdoors Essentials checklist on the next page to help you with your planning.

Wilderness Survival Gear

Because of the risks associated with injury and weather, remote wilderness trips are not recommended during pregnancy, especially after the first trimester. Injuries as a result of falls or extreme temperature exposure are serious risks during pregnancy, both for the mother and the fetus. But if you do decide to head into the wilderness, even if just for the day, you should be prepared to handle rapidly changing weather, getting lost, signaling in case of an emergency, and surviving for a few days on your own. Remain within cell phone or signaling distance of help, let someone know where you are going and when you plan to return, and don't go alone. Before you leave, pack a lightweight and portable survival kit to take with you, just in case.

Outdoors Essentials

- ☐ Backpack
- ☐ Bandanna
- ☐ Cell phone
- ☐ Compass
- ☐ Identification
- ☐ Insect repellent
- ☐ Lip balm
- ☐ Map
- ☐ Plastic bag (for trash)
- ☐ Pocket knife
- ☐ Sunglasses
- ☐ Sunscreen
- ☐ Toilet paper
- ☐ Watch
- ☐ Water (16 ounces per hour)
- ☐ Waterproof matches

CLOTHING

- ☐ Breathable jacket
- ☐ Extra socks
- ☐ Gloves
- ☐ Long-sleeved shirt
- ☐ Rain gear and hood
- ☐ Sun hat
- ☐ Swimsuit

EXTRAS

- ☐ Binoculars
- ☐ Camera
- ☐ Extra batteries
- ☐ Field guide
- ☐ First aid kit and manual
- ☐ Flashlight
- ☐ Reading glasses

FOOD

- ☐ Dried fruit and nuts
- ☐ Energy bars
- ☐ Granola bars
- ☐ Powdered drinks
- ☐ Sandwiches

Whether you are going around the block or into the backcountry, good preparation is essential when you are expecting. If you pick your gear carefully, you should be comfortable and feel safe heading outdoors during pregnancy.

Emergency Survival Kit

- ☐ Aluminum foil
- ☐ Blaze orange smoke signal
- ☐ Bouillon cubes
- ☐ Candle
- ☐ Compass
- ☐ Energy bars
- ☐ Flashlight

- ☐ Magnesium fire starter
- ☐ Signal mirror
- ☐ Space blanket
- ☐ Sugar and salt packets
- ☐ Tea bags
- ☐ Water-purification tablets or water filter
- ☐ Whistle (to call for help)

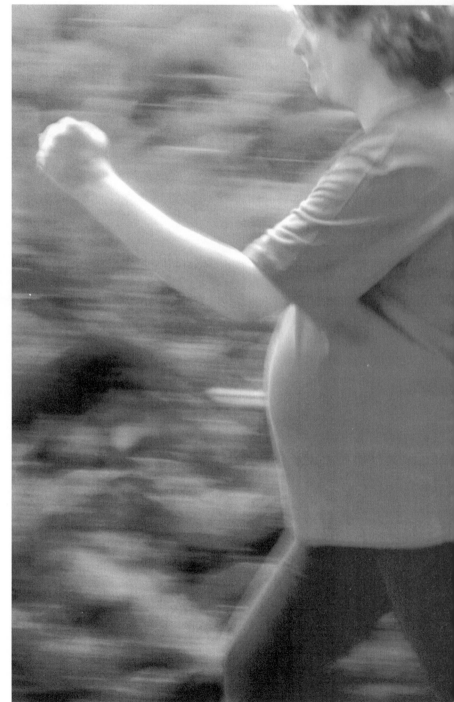

chapter **5**

FIRST AID BASICS

• • •

**PACKING A
PREGNANCY-SAFE
FIRST AID KIT**

First Aid and Preventive Gear for Pregnancy

As an active mother-to-be, you probably already recognize the importance of good preventive gear. With the help of your handy first aid kit, you can avoid a blistering sunburn, banish a swarm of annoying insects, and even handle a minor injury like a pro. During pregnancy, you may have to make some adjustments so that your trusted first aid kit, sunscreen, insect repellent, and water purifier are safe for your fetus too.

First Aid Basics

As you put together your first aid kit, keep in mind that small and portable is best. A plastic box that seals shut or a waterproof bag works well. Take care to label everything carefully and clearly.

Protection from Sun and Heat

Sunscreen will be the thing from your first aid kit that you use most frequently. You should apply sunscreen everyday. Use sunscreen even if you are indoors, in the shade, or outdoors on a cloudy day. Remember that sun reflects strongly off water, sand, and snow. Wind (especially if your skin becomes wind-burned) can also make a sunburn worse.

How to Prevent Sunburn and Overheating

- Avoid exercise during hot and humid weather.

- Stay out of hot tubs and saunas.

- Dress in removable layers of light-colored clothing that covers all sun-exposed skin.

- Use sunscreen (SPF 30 or above) every day.

- Wear a hat and sunglasses to protect your face and eyes.

- Exercise during cooler times of the day and take frequent breaks in the shade.

- Drink at least one liter of water per hour of exercise. If it is very hot, try sports drinks to replace your salts (electrolytes) and keep you better hydrated.

- Avoid caffeinated (and alcoholic) drinks, since these increase fluid loss.

- Exercise at a slower pace to keep your heart rate lower, so you can stay cool.

- If you suspect that you are too hot, check your underarm temperature: it should be below 101°F.

- If outside temperatures rise suddenly—as at the beginning of summer—take a few days to get used to the heat before you start exercising at all.

Even without going out in the sun, you may have noticed that you have that special glow of pregnancy. Increased blood flow to the skin during pregnancy causes that characteristic blush—and it also makes you more likely to burn. You've probably seen some other skin changes as well, such as darkening of your nipples, areolae (the darker skin right around your nipples), belly button, vulva, and armpits. Some women even develop a blotchy rash across their forehead, cheeks, and nose, which is called *melasma* or the "mask of pregnancy," and can look like a bad sunburn. Melasma is not caused by sun exposure, but going out in the sun can make it look a lot worse. The sun can also exaggerate other skin changes, like dark skin spots and spider veins. If you weren't motivated to protect your skin before, maybe those highlighted veins will convince you. Just a little sunscreen will do the trick.

Sunscreen creams and lotions help block the sun's ultraviolet rays that burn your skin. The SPF (sun protection factor) of the sunscreen indicates its actual protection value: the higher the SPF, the better the burn protection. If you have dark skin or rarely burn, SPF 15 should be the minimum protection you use. For longer exposure or fair skin, SPF 30 or higher sunscreen is safer. If you will be on the water or in direct sunlight, opaque sunscreens, such as those with zinc oxide, may protect your skin even better.

Since you sweat more during pregnancy, a waterproof sunscreen is a good choice. Put on sunscreen before insect repellent and under thin clothing. The chemicals in sunscreen are safe for use during pregnancy, so don't hesitate to use plenty.

In addition to protecting your skin from the sun, you should watch out for very hot and humid weather. If you feel sweaty and worn out or if it's steaming outside, just cancel your plans and stay indoors. You are more susceptible to heat exhaustion during pregnancy, so keep a tall glass of ice water at your side, stay in a cool place, rest, and try placing a moist towel on your neck and forehead. Think about it this way: the more comfortable you are, the more comfortable your fetus will be.

Protection from Cold and Wind

Chances are you'll worry more about going out in the cold when you're holding your baby in your arms—now, you're probably inclined to just shiver and bear it. Your body does a good job of keeping your fetus warm even when you are freezing. Nonetheless, you should bundle up during pregnancy.

Why? Because you lose a lot of your heat by sweating more and because of your greater surface area (that big belly loses a lot of warmth) when you're pregnant. If you are also worn out, stressed, or dehydrated, you may be more vulnerable to cold illness, or hypothermia. Exposing your fingers and toes to the cold can give you frostnip (which affects just the surface of the skin) or frostbite (which can involve the full thickness of skin and underlying tissues). So take those cold-weather woolies and layer up if you're going to be outside in the cold for more than a few minutes. If you feel chilly, bundle up and keep moving— exercise can help you keep your core warm and prevent cold illness and frostbite. Hot chocolate and apple cider also work wonders.

How to Prevent Cold Injury and Illness

- Check weather reports (not just for town but also for the top of the mountain) to get a good sense of conditions during the day and at night.

- Wear layers: the more layers of clothing, the better the insulation.

- Wear a windproof and water-repellent outer shell.

- Choose wool, polypropylene, and pile fabrics to wear closer to the skin, since these trap warm air and do not collapse when wet.

- Wear a hat, scarf, thick socks, mittens, and gloves to keep yourself toasty.

- To prevent frostbite, smooth out wrinkles in socks, avoid lacing shoes too tightly, and choose well-fitting boots so that you maintain good circulation to your feet.

- In very cold or windy weather or if you're skiing, wear a mask and goggles to protect your face, since windchill affects exposed skin.

- Carry snacks and plenty of fluids. Hunger and dehydration make cold illness, or hypothermia, worse.

- If the weather changes, do not hesitate to head home early.

- Keep your spirits up! Feeling depressed increases your risk of cold illness.

Remember, the cold can be deceiving: you may be sweaty after exercising, but you still need to keep yourself insulated if it's cold, wet, or windy. And be prepared for rapid changes in weather, especially in the fall or spring or if you live in an area that is prone to thundershowers. You could be in trouble if you are hiking in a t-shirt and get caught in a sudden hailstorm.

Protection from Insect Bites and Infections

You may have noticed that you've gotten more insect bites during pregnancy. Why? First, you are sweating more and have a lot of blood at your skin surface—just what insects are looking for. Second, bites cause a more severe inflammatory reaction in pregnancy, meaning bites are more visible and they itch more.

Most insect bites are simply annoying. But some bites, like that of a Lyme disease–infected tick or a malaria-carrying mosquito, can cause illness. If you are exercising around your city neighborhood, chances are you won't even have

INSECT-BORNE ILLNESS	TYPE OF BUG	REGION WHERE TYPICALLY FOUND
Babesiosis	Parasite carried by tick	North America
Colorado Tick Fever	Virus carried by ticks	Colorado (especially March to October)
Dengue Fever	Virus carried by mosquitoes	Africa, Caribbean, Mexico, South America, Southeast Asia
Ehrlichiosis	Bacteria carried by ticks	North America
Lyme Disease	Bacteria carried by ticks	Asia, Australia, Canada, Europe, Russia, North America (especially summer and early fall)
Malaria	Bacteria carried by mosquitoes	Central and South America, Middle East, Southeast Asia, sub-Saharan Africa
Relapsing Fever	Bacteria carried by ticks	Canada, western U.S.A.
Rocky Mountain Spotted Fever	Bacteria carried by ticks	Southeastern U.S.A. and Texas (especially late spring to summer)
Tularemia	Bacteria carried by ticks and contaminated water	North America
West Nile Fever	Virus carried by mosquitoes	Africa, Eastern Europe, Middle East, South America, U.S.A.
Yellow Fever	Virus carried by mosquitoes	Central and South America, tropical and west Africa

to think about insect-borne illness. Insects that carry disease are rare in urban areas in the United States.

You can talk with your doctor or check the Centers for Disease Control (CDC) website (www.cdc.gov) to learn what insects and illnesses exist in a specific area. The table on the previous page gives you some idea of common insect-borne diseases and where may be found.

If you do get bitten and the itching is driving you crazy, try applying a topical anesthetic cream, or 1-percent hydrocortisone cream to decrease the inflammation. But, if you take a few simple precautions, you can simply avoid getting bitten in the first place.

Clearly, choosing not to use insect repellent can be risky for both you and your fetus, since insects can carry dangerous disease. However, unlike sunscreen, some insect repellents can also pose a risk to your fetus. Because you are probably trying to avoid harmful chemicals, finding a safe insect repellent may seem somewhat intimidating.

You have many choices when selecting an insect repellent. The best option for you depends on your risks of insect exposure. For example, in an area with tick-transmitted Lyme disease, using a repellent that is effective against ticks is very important. For a short summer walk in your neighborhood park, a short-acting repellent that works on a variety of annoying insects may be sufficient.

Natural repellents, including citronella and lemon eucalyptus, are safe during pregnancy but are not very effective against most insects. They typically offer you some protection for one to two hours and are best used in areas where insects are somewhat irritating but don't carry disease.

Synthetic repellents, such as those with DEET, are extremely effective, widely used, and considered safe for use during pregnancy. Apply synthetic repellents directly to the skin, avoiding broken skin and the areas near the lips and eyes where you may experience a toxic reaction. You can also use DEET repellent on your clothing, but it may damage some synthetic fabrics, such as polyester and leather.

When these repellents are applied to the skin, some DEET is absorbed through the skin and enters your circulation. For safey, pick a repellent with a concentration of less than 33 percent DEET. To minimize absorption through the skin, choose extended-release DEET-based repellents, which have lower DEET concentrations and offer longer-lasting protection.

How to Prevent Insect Bites, Stings, and Insect-Borne Illness

- Wear lightweight, long-sleeved shirts with fitted cuffs.

- Wear long socks and tuck pants into them, especially at dusk and dawn.

- Choose light-colored fabrics, such as pastels, which attract fewer insects than dark colors.

- Avoid using perfumes or scented soaps, which can attract insects.

- At the end of the day, inspect your entire body for ticks, including your armpits and groin.

- If you are spending the night outdoors, use mosquito netting or a tent. Choose a site away from stagnant water, restrooms, and other areas where insects congregate.

- In areas with insect-borne disease, spray tent and clothing with permethrin insect repellent.

- Put up and seal the net or tent before high insect-activity periods, such as sunset. Before sleeping, vigilantly clear your tent of insects.

- Apply sunscreen before applying your insect repellent.

- Apply insect repellents (with 20 to 33 percent DEET if there is a risk of insect-borne disease) to exposed skin, avoiding broken skin and the areas around the lips and eyes.

- If you have had a serious reaction to an insect bite or sting in the past, talk to your doctor about carrying a self-injectable epinephrine kit in case of a life-threatening reaction and wear a medical alert bracelet that identifies you as allergic to insect stings.

- Use caution when in areas with potential insect hazards, such as anthills, wasp nests, or spider hiding places—your best protection is not to disturb them!

Insecticides are the third category of repellents. Permethrin insecticides are safe for use during pregnancy because you apply them to your clothing or bedding, not directly on your skin. You can use permethrin on your tents, mosquito nets, or sleeping bags without damaging the fabrics. It will continue to repel insects for weeks or months—even after multiple washings. Permethrin is very effective against chiggers, ticks, mosquitoes, fleas, and sand flies and it helps prevent malaria when sprayed on netting.

When you are gardening, avoid applying pesticides, insecticides, and fertilizers yourself, and handle treated plants with gloves. Many studies show that these chemicals can be absorbed through the skin and may harm the developing fetus. Organic compost is not free of risks either. Working with rotting wood or soil can cause fungal infections. Inhaling dust while outdoors can also transmit some infections, such as coccidioidomycosis (also called "valley fever" or "desert rheumatism") in the western United States. This infection can become quite serious—even fatal—if untreated, especially during the third trimester of pregnancy. Also, watch out for puncture wounds or scratches from rose thorns, straw, mosses, or wood splinters, which can cause sporotrichosis, a fungal infection.

Protection from Unsafe Water

If you are active, you know how important drinking water is for your health. If you haven't been drinking enough, you'll feel worn out and weak. And if you don't catch up on your fluids, you can become quite ill. If you're heading out into the wilderness or to a developing country, you should make sure your drinking water

WATER-BORNE ILLNESS	TYPE OF BUG	REGION WHERE TYPICALLY FOUND
Campylobacter	Bacteria on farm animals in raw milk, or in contaminated water	North America
Cryptosporidium	Parasites in contaminated water	North America
Giardia	Parasites in contaminated water	North America
Leptospirosis	Water contaminated by infected animal urine	North America
Schistosomiasis	Parasitic flatworms in freshwater snails	Africa, Asia, Caribbean islands, Middle East, South America
Typhoid Fever	Bacteria in contaminated food or water	Africa, Asia

How to Prevent Dehydration and Water-Borne Illness During Pregnancy

- Keep drinking water handy. Drink up even if you don't feel thirsty and even if you're just sitting around.

- Nothing beats water to keep you hydrated—drink juices, sodas, and sports drinks only occasionally.

- If in doubt, treat the water. Consider all outdoor water supplies possible sources of water-borne illness and contaminants.

- If you're heading out for the day, carry water (one liter per person per hour) with you and pack iodine water purification tablets in case you run out.

is safe. Tap water abroad may not be well purified. Similarly, in the back-country, you cannot assume that clear running water is safe to drink. Surface water can carry a risk of intestinal illness due to bacteria, viruses, and protozoan cysts—such as *Giardia lamblia*, the most common contaminant in North American wilderness water. In the table on the previous page, I outline some common water-borne illnesses and where they are found.

Drinking unpurified water can give you a terrible case of diarrhea and vomiting and make you dangerously dehydrated. It's worth the hassle to port around bottles of safe water, carry a filter, or put up with the taste of water treatment tablets.

On a day trip, you can probably manage to lug around enough water to meet your needs. But if you don't carry all your water with you, you'll need to disinfect any stream or creek water you find *before* you drink it. There are several ways to purify water and the best method during pregnancy depends on the local risks and the length of time you will be drinking the treated water.

Heat disinfection is very effective in killing disease-causing microorganisms and is a safe method of purifying drinking water during pregnancy, especially in the wilderness. Bringing water to a boil (212°F at sea level), even at high altitude, where water boils at lower temperatures, disinfects it. Boil very polluted water for a minute or bring to a boil then leave covered for several minutes. However, surprisingly, bringing to a boil is not essential—heating to 140°F for thirty minutes is also effective. Keep in mind that heat disinfection does not get rid of chemical contaminants, which may be present in a stream where there is a mine, a city, or factories upstream. Heat disinfection is the recommended method of preventing water-borne illness.

Water filters for the wilderness are able to remove protozoa like *Giardia* and intestinal bacteria but may not remove the much smaller viruses that can also cause disease. Higher-quality water filters incorporate an iodine resin to kill viruses and an activated charcoal filter to absorb chemical contaminants in the water. These combination filters are very effective in making high-risk water safe. However, iodine remains in the water, making it unsafe for continuous use for longer than three weeks during pregnancy.

Clarification techniques, such as adding aluminum sulfate and filtering, sedimentation (allowing the water to stand for an hour and pouring off the clear portion), and charcoal purifiers, remove suspended particles in cloudy water and improve taste, but these methods do not disinfect the water. The water may look clear, but it may not be safe, especially for a pregnant woman. To make the water potable after clarifying, you must treat it with a combination filter or heat disinfect it.

Iodine kills microorganisms and binds with chemical impurities in the water, making them inactive. However, iodine is not effective against a protozoal organism called *Cryptosporidium*, which does not pose much of a risk in North American alpine areas but presents a much greater risk in lowland rivers and developing countries. Do not rely on iodine tablets or chlorine to purify water in areas that may have towns or camps upstream, since *Cryptosporidium* can make you very ill and endanger your pregnancy.

Iodine water purification tablets or crystals are easy to use and carry but should not be used to purify water for longer than three weeks during pregnancy. This is because iodine remains active in the body, affects the fetus, and can be toxic in high doses. Using "neutralizing tablets" (ascorbic acid) after the iodine tablets to improve the color and taste does not remove the active iodine. Instead, it just converts the iodine to iodide, which still affects the body—and the fetus. Nonpregnant users can drink iodine-purified water safely for a few months.

Chlorination and dechlorination with peroxide is efficient for disinfecting large quantities of water. The chlorine becomes tasteless calcium chloride during the process. Chlorine-purified water is considered safe throughout pregnancy with no time limit on use. However, a pregnant woman should not handle the high-concentration chlorine (calcium hypochlorite) crystals or the corrosive 30-percent hydrogen peroxide solution used in the disinfecting process.

Remember that all water collected outdoors, including spring water, dew, snowmelt, and pond ice, needs to be disinfected. During pregnancy, heat disinfection (preceded by clarification or filtration) is the preferred method, since it is nontoxic and highly effective. For short trips into the wilderness (or into developing countries), combination filters with iodine resin and charcoal filters are convenient and effective. For a day trip, carry iodine water purification tablets in your pack in case of an emergency—during pregnancy, clean water is a fundamental safety concern.

Packing a Pregnancy-Safe First Aid Kit

It is a good idea to put together a first aid kit containing pregnancy-safe medications in case of an emergency. Your first aid kit will also help you deal with minor problems such as nausea and skin scrapes. This may be a kit that you keep in your car or in a readily accessible place in your home. You may use it long after your baby is born. And if you are heading outdoors for more than a couple of hours, consider packing a small first aid travel kit to keep in your backpack too.

Some medicines are approved by the U.S. Food and Drug Administration (FDA) for use during pregnancy; these are considered safe for you and the fetus. But when you are pregnant, you should avoid using unnecessary and unsafe medications. Consider using alternatives to medications to treat common problems, such as drinking ginger tea to reduce nausea or firmly squeezing the fleshy area between your thumb and forefinger to ease a headache.

Unsafe Medications

If you already have a first aid kit at home, make sure that you know what medications you can use safely during pregnancy. Many medicines have simply not been tested on pregnant women and should only be used if absolutely necessary. If your doctor recommends a medication, she probably feels that the benefits of taking the medication outweigh the possible risks. But don't hesitate to talk to your doctor if you have any concerns about the medications she prescribes.

A few medications that are commonly found in first aid kits are not considered completely safe during pregnancy or are not safe during certain trimesters

Unsafe Medications for Pregnancy: Take These Out of Your First Aid Kit

Pain and Inflammation Medications

- **Aspirin (Ecotrin, Bayer, ASA)**
- **Ibuprofen (Advil, Motrin, Nuprin)**
- **Naproxen (Naprosyn, Aleve, Anaprox)**

Decongestant Medications

- **Diphenhydramine (Benadryl, Allerdryl)**
- **Oxymetazoline (Afrin, Dristan, Nostrilla)**
- **Phenylephrine (Neo-Synephrine, Sinex, Nostril)**
- **Pseudoephedrine (Sudafed, Allegra, Actifed, Detussin)**
- **Triamcinolone (Nasacort)**

Nausea and Vomiting Medications

- **Prochlorperazine (Compazine)**
- **Promethazine (Phenergan)**

Motion Sickness Medication

- **Scopolamine (Transderm Scop)**

Cough Medications

- **Benzonatate (Tessalon Perles)**
- **Guaifenesin (Robitussin DM, Robitussin AC, Robitussin PE, Hytuss, Guiatuss)**

Diarrhea Medications

- **Bismuth Subsalicylate (Pepto Bismol)**
- **Diphenoxylate (Lomotil)**

Antibiotic Ointments

- **Bacitracin**
- **Neosporin**
- **Polysporin**

(for example, diphenhydramine, commonly marketed as Benadryl, is not safe during your first trimester but can be taken during your second or third trimesters). Remove these potentially unsafe medications from your family's first aid kit or label them clearly so you don't use them by mistake. The chart above gives you the generic and brand names of unsafe medications during pregnancy.

First Aid Checklist

So now you know what medications to remove from your existing first aid kit. If you need to put together a pregnancy-safe first aid kit, here is a basic checklist. You only need small amounts of each item—just replace them as you use them—since you'll want to keep the kit small and portable. Label the pill containers carefully.

Your Pregnancy-Safe First Aid Kit

Medications

- **FOR ACID REFLUX: calcium carbonate (Tums, Rolaids)**
- **FOR CONGESTION: saline nasal spray (SeaMist, NaSal)**
- **FOR COUGH: dextromethorphan (Vicks, Benylin, Delsym)**
- **FOR DIARRHEA: attapulgite (Kaopectate, Diasorb)**
- **FOR HEMORRHOIDS: pramoxine (Anusol) or witch hazel (Tucks)**
- **FOR ITCH: calamine lotion or oatmeal cream (Aveeno)**
- **FOR MOTION SICKNESS: dimenhydrinate (Dramamine)**
- **FOR NAUSEA OR VOMITING: doxylamine (Unisom Sleep Aid)**
- **FOR PAIN OR FEVER: acetaminophen (Tylenol)**

Wound Care

- **Aloe vera gel**
- **Antiseptic towelettes**
- **Bandage strips**
- **Elastic cloth bandage to wrap sprained joints**
- **Moleskin to prevent blisters**
- **Povidone-iodine solution**
- **Safety pins**
- **Sterile gauze pads**
- **Tape**

Equipment

- **Latex or vinyl exam gloves**
- **Small notebook and pencil**
- **Small scissors**
- **Thermometer**
- **Tweezers**
- **Waterproof first aid box**

Safety Gear

- **Insect repellent**
- **Lip balm with sunscreen**
- **Sunscreen (SPF 30 or greater)**

Preparing your first aid and safety gear ahead of time will make it easy for you to stay active and safe during pregnancy. Whether you are camping or gardening, having some basic first aid materials nearby is very useful—and a good practice for when you become a parent too.

chapter 6

A HEALTHY WARM-UP

• • •

DYNAMIC STRETCHING
TO PREVENT INJURY

• • •

MONITORING
YOUR EXERCISE

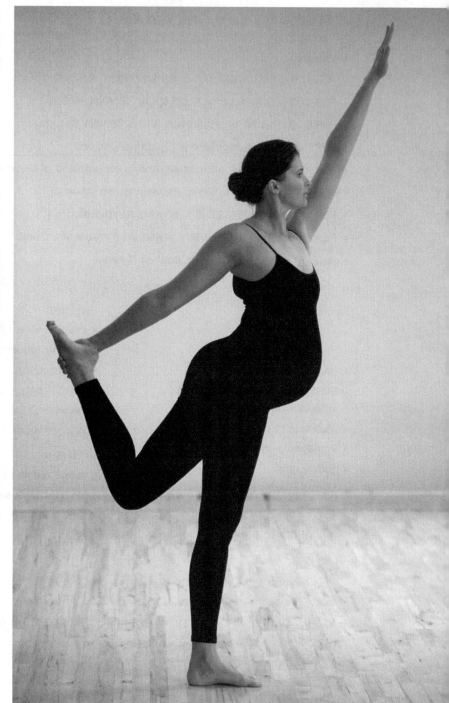

Warming Up and Monitoring Your Exercise

If you have ever suffered a muscle strain while exercising, you know the importance of warming up before working out. The warm-up is essential during pregnancy, when your relaxed ligaments, increased weight, and shifted center of gravity may make injuries more painful. Exercising rigorously without warming up can also affect the blood flow to your fetus. So if you're short on time, skip the workout, but don't skip the warm-up.

A Healthy Warm-Up

Warming up activates your muscles and heart, gradually shifting the body's focus from its resting tasks, such as digesting and storing energy, to active tasks, such as movement and burning energy. Exercise forces the bulk of your blood to your muscles and skin. As your muscles start to work, they need more oxygen and nutrients and increased blood flow to clear away the toxins created by exercise. If you exert yourself without warming up, your muscles don't get that extra circulation immediately, and you feel a cramp—caused by the buildup of one of those toxins, called lactic acid.

Because exercising abruptly (sprinting or racing, for example) pulls blood away from your internal organs, including your uterus, the fetus may experience decreased blood flow and oxygen for a brief period. However, if you begin to exercise slowly with a good warm-up, your heart and lungs have a chance to rev up and maintain adequate blood flow to the uterus and to your fetus.

For at least five minutes before you start exercising, do some light activity to gently stimulate the circulation in your muscles. In cold weather, if you are injured, or right after waking up, take a little more time to warm up. The best warm-up activity is a targeted warm-up, an easy version of what you plan to do next that activates the muscle groups you will be using. For example, if you will be running, skiing, or snowshoeing, try walking for five or ten minutes first. If you plan to swim, snorkel, or surf, try swimming a few easy lengths.

Dynamic Stretching to Prevent Injury

After you have warmed up, try a few dynamic stretches, which are smooth movements that improve the flexibility of your muscles, improve their blood flow, and prepare you for exercise. Dynamic stretches should expand the range of motion (how far you can comfortably stretch) of the specific muscle groups and joints you will use while exercising. These stretches are different from the static stretches you do to relax after working out, where you stretch a muscle and hold the position. As with all exercise, if the stretch doesn't feel comfortable, stop and rest.

Activate your abdominal and buttocks muscles by lying on your back with your knees bent, your feet flat on the ground, and your arms lying alongside your body. Then tighten your abdominals, squeeze your buttocks, and lift your hips upward slowly. You will feel the tension through your belly and hips and in your buttocks. Then slowly lower your hips back to the ground. Between repetitions, roll to your left side to avoid becoming light-headed while lying on your back. Repeat the hip lift ten times and do three sets of ten, increasing the height of your hips with each set.

Activate your back by getting on your hands and knees and doing a cat stretch: pull in your abdominals, round up your spine, and gently tuck your hips and pelvis under you. Then relax and flatten your back until it is parallel to the ground again. Repeat, doing two sets of ten stretches.

Activate your hips by standing with your feet shoulder-width apart and moving your hips in a gentle circle. Keep your feet still and your back straight while you rotate one direction for ten circles and then the opposite direction for ten.

Activate your legs by doing supported squats. Stand facing a table or other sturdy support with your hands on the table and your feet shoulder-width apart. Squat down as if you are sitting in an invisible chair, keeping your back straight, abdominals tucked in, and knees over your toes. Squat only as low as you are comfortable and can easily get up, since the weight of your pregnancy adds resistance. Exhale as you use your thigh muscles to return to standing. Do two sets of ten squats.

Activate your neck by tilting your head from side to side, ear to shoulder, ten times. Then gently drop your neck forward and roll toward one shoulder then the other, in half circles, ten times.

Activate your shoulders by doing shoulder shrugs, bringing your shoulders up near your ears, then rotating them forward and down. Relax, then repeat the shrug. Do ten forward shrugs, then ten backward shrugs, rotating the shoulders back and down.

Activate your arms by doing arm circles. Standing with your feet shoulder-width apart and your back upright, hold your arms straight out from your sides. Rotate your arms in little circles ten times going forward, then ten times going backward. Perform three sets in each direction, making bigger arm circles with each set.

Monitoring Your Exercise

It is healthy to stay in good shape during pregnancy, but remember that your goal is to have a healthy pregnancy—not to push yourself to build muscle mass, lose weight, or exercise competitively. Sweating too much, crashing after a killer workout, and working out until your entire body aches are simply not healthy for your pregnancy. If you feel overtired, unable to continue exercising, or are in pain, modify your routine. Build in breaks to release your muscles and hydrate while exercising. As you exercise, assess your level of exertion so that you know you are getting a healthy workout, but not pushing yourself too hard. You'll do this by keeping an eye on your heart rate, your breathing, and your hydration.

Monitoring Your Heart Rate

As you exercise, your heart works harder to deliver blood—with its oxygen and nutrients—to your muscles as well as other important organs of your body: your brain, your skin, your lungs, and, of course, your uterus. The harder you work out, the harder your heart pumps. As you do so, you are conditioning your heart—and perhaps your fetus's heart as well—to work more efficiently. This is why well-conditioned athletes have lower resting heart rates: their hearts pump more blood with each beat.

Getting your heart pumping when you head outdoors is good for you. However, you want to make sure you aren't pushing your heart too hard. If you feel like you are working very hard, slow down. Even moderate exertion will get you in better shape. Remember that the pregnancy puts extra strain on your heart, so your heart rate during pregnancy is higher than usual to start with.

You'll want to monitor your heart rate during the most strenuous part of your workout. Slow your pace so that you can take your pulse. It is easiest to feel your pulse on the inside of your wrist or on the side of your neck. Turn your hand so the palm is up and use the index and middle fingers on your other hand to locate your pulse on the thumb side of your wrist. Or feel the pulse on either side of your Adam's apple, on your neck. Press gently so you feel every beat and count the beats for fifteen seconds. Multiply this number by four to get your number of beats per minute—this is your heart rate. During exercise, your heart rate should stay below 145 beats per minute (a good workout is 100 to 140 beats per minute). If your heart rate is above this level, slow down, hydrate, and continue more cautiously. If your heart rate is less than 100 beats per minute, pick up your pace so that you get a better workout!

Monitoring Your Breathing

Your breathing will also give you a good sense of how much you are exerting yourself. As you work your muscles, your lungs need to deliver more oxygen and get rid of more carbon dioxide—so you breath harder. Taking deep, rapid breaths increases the space for clean air in your lungs; the harder you work, the more air your lungs move in and out. During pregnancy, your body needs more oxygen in general because your metabolism is revved up and your fetus depends on your lungs for its oxygen. Plus, as your belly grows, it puts pressure on your diaphragm making you feel as if you can't take really deep breaths. So you may feel out of breath even with minor exercise during pregnancy.

If you are out of breath, you should slow down. The easiest way to monitor your breathing is to make sure you are comfortable talking while exercising. If you can't carry on a conversation, you are pushing yourself too hard.

Monitoring Your Hydration

As soon as your body warms up when you are exercising, you start to lose fluids by sweating and by breathing with your mouth open. You can become dehydrated very quickly especially in hot weather, if you are overdressed, if you exercise longer or harder than usual, if you are ill, or have a fever. Dehydration is very dangerous during pregnancy because, among other things, it can cause you to overheat or develop preterm contractions—both of which are potentially dangerous for your fetus.

In general, you should make sure you are drinking at least a liter of water per hour outdoors, even if you don't feel thirsty. Drink more if it is hot, you are exerting yourself, or you feel thirsty. Hydrate well before beginning exercise and carry water with you—even on a neighborhood walk—or bring gear to purify water in the wilderness. If you exercise for more than two or three hours, you will also need to replace your salts by eating snacks and drinking sports drinks or rehydration fluids with electrolytes (salts).

Look out for signs of dehydration: dry mouth and lips, decreased sweating, pale skin, headache, fatigue, muscle cramps, or contractions. You should need to urinate at least every four hours and your urine should be light yellow. If it is dark yellow or less frequent, you are dehydrated already. Slow down and hydrate.

Monitoring your exertion while you are active is just as important to your health as warming up and cooling down. It will also give you a good sense of how your heart and lungs are getting better conditioned as you exercise regularly.

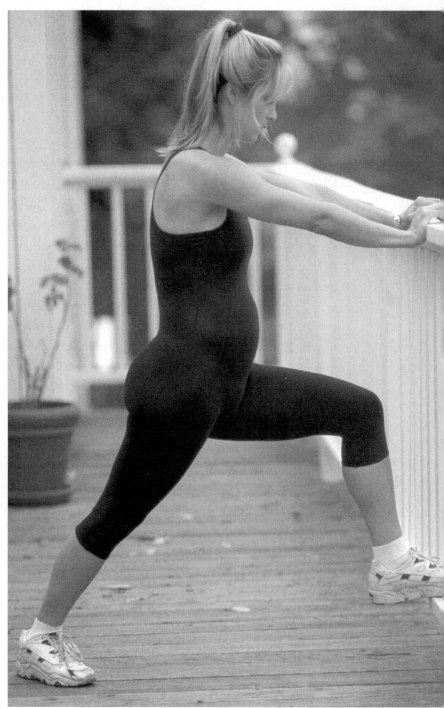

chapter 7

A HEALTHY BREAK

• • •

COOLING DOWN

• • •

STRETCHES FOR PREGNANCY

Taking Breaks, Cooling Down, and Stretching

When you exercise during pregnancy, you will find that you become tired more easily and need to take breaks more frequently. Listen to your body and slow down before you feel too worn out or achy. Taking breaks properly can prevent fatigue, soreness, and joint pain.

Cooling down and stretching also prevents post-exercise discomfort. A healthy workout includes a cooldown period too. Use the last ten minutes of your exercise time to improve flexibility and gently transition blood flow back to your internal organs. Cooling down pays off in the long run, since you'll feel more resilient—and more likely to exercise regularly.

A Healthy Break

The number one rule for taking breaks is: Take them. Many active women forget to tone down their activities once they are pregnant even though their bodies are working much harder to support the pregnancy. Your heart, lungs, and muscles all work overtime to nurture your growing body and fetus, and a workout only adds to that strain. As your pregnancy progresses, it is normal to need breaks during the course of a regular working day. The tips described here apply to all breaks—on the trail, on the beach, and even at home or in the office.

Use your breaks to drink water, eat small snacks, release your muscles, and catch your breath. If you are doing rigorous exercise, try doing a few stretches as you rest to loosen your muscles—like shoulder shrugs, flexing your toes, and stretching your arms. Remember to look around you and enjoy the outdoors while you're at it—feeling relaxed and peaceful is also important for a healthy pregnancy.

Being tired will make your outdoor activities less fun and will make you more vulnerable to certain problems, such as heat exhaustion, altitude illness, cold illness (hypothermia), muscle strain, and falls. The best prevention is to plan an excursion that is reasonable for your pregnant body and take frequent breaks.

Use your breaks to assess how you feel. If you have lots of energy left and feel great, you may choose to continue your activity. If you are starting to feel worn out, take the opportunity to discuss an alternative plan (or a route home) so you don't push yourself too hard.

Ask yourself a few questions:

- Do I feel any contractions or cramps?

- Is my baby moving less than usual—even when I am resting?

- Have I been urinating less than once every four hours?

- Do I have any worrisome symptoms? Headache? Light-headedness? Shortness of breath? Muscle or joint pain? Feeling unwell?

- Am I becoming tired?

If your answer is "yes" to any of these questions—or if you simply don't feel like continuing the activity—let your companions know that you need to stop and get back home.

Getting Off Your Feet

Most important, get off your feet for a few minutes during your break. This is not always as easy as it sounds, since if you're hiking or swimming you probably won't have a couch to flop onto. If you are outdoors, you'll need to take a few things into consideration when getting off your feet during pregnancy. Your balance is off, so lean against something while sitting down or getting up. After your second trimester, your uterus is large enough that you may find it difficult to get up once you do sit down—sitting on a bench (or a fallen tree) is easier than sitting on the ground. Make yourself comfortable, even if it's only for a few minutes.

While you're giving your feet a rest, you may slouch and injure your back, ultimately making yourself more tired. Maintain good posture, whether you are sitting, lying down, or standing.

Healthy Posture for Sitting. Try to find a bench where you can sit with the length of your thighs supported. You will find that you are more comfortable on a seat with good back support than on a cozy chair. Sit with your knees level with your hips and avoid slouching. Tuck your pelvis under you so that your back is not arched and your ears, shoulders, and hips are aligned. It may help to place a rolled towel behind your buttocks to support the small of your back. Don't cross your legs, since this can decrease the circulation to your legs—leading to leg swelling and a risk of blood clots.

If you must sit on the ground, sit upright, with your legs bent but not crossed—sitting cross-legged during pregnancy can strain your back. If you have pain in your tailbone (the coccyx), sit on a cushion. If you can, lean against a firm vertical surface and place a rolled towel behind your buttocks. A pillow placed under your knees will also keep your pelvis tucked under you and help keep your back aligned, preventing back pain.

Healthy Posture for Lying Down. You can take a rejuvenating break and also give your back a rest if you lie down on a firm, cushioned surface, whether it is a bed or a sleeping pad. Don't lie down immediately after exercising, since putting your head at the level of your heart may make you light-headed. Cool off, sit, hydrate, then lie down.

Remember that lying flat on your back or on your right side for long periods after your first trimester (especially after about twenty weeks) is not healthy because the weight of your uterus can decrease your circulation. If you lie on your left side, your placenta and fetus get maximal blood flow because the uterus is not putting pressure on the major blood vessels and you take the strain off your legs and back. When you lie on your side, you may want to place a pillow behind you to support your back and a pillow under your belly to support the weight of your uterus. You can also decrease lower back strain and help distribute the weight of the upper leg by putting a pillow between your bent knees.

Staying semireclined is also healthy for the pregnancy. In this position, support your back with pillows, elevate your head, and keep your knees bent.

You may want to put a pillow or a rolled towel under your knees so that your back is not arched.

To get up, roll all the way over to one side, keeping your knees together, and use your arms to slowly push yourself to a sitting position. Sit for a few moments to avoid light-headedness before you stand up. Then, keeping your back straight and your head up, tuck your legs under you and stand up using your thigh muscles.

Healthy Posture for Standing. Even if you are standing for long periods, you can still give your legs a rest by shifting your weight. Put one foot up on a step or low stool—this helps reduce the arch in your lower back. In addition, tuck your pelvis under you by gently tightening your buttocks and abdominal muscles so that your back and neck are straight, with your ears, shoulders, and hips in line.

While standing, you can release some of the tension in your back and bring the weight of your uterus closer to your center of gravity—while improving your posture—by doing a pelvic tilt. Practice this motion by standing with your back to a wall, sliding your hand into the hollow of your back, and tilting your pelvis forward so that your lower back is pressed firmly against your hand and the wall. Hold this position for a few seconds, then slowly release.

Taking frequent breaks will help you maintain your energy level and allow you to check in with your body. When you start up after your break, take it slowly for a few minutes; warm up before doing anything more strenuous, since your body's already working twice as hard during pregnancy.

Cooling Down

One of the most gratifying and relaxing parts of a workout is the cool down, when your rapid heart rate subsides and you release the muscles that have been working so hard. Cooling down is essential during pregnancy because it helps your body maintain blood flow to the fetus and strengthens your ligaments and joints, which are prone to injury. Take time to cool down before you eat or crash in the easy chair after exercise—even if you were just mowing the lawn—you'll feel better and you and your fetus will be healthier.

A healthy cooldown has three components: gently lowering the intensity of exercise and allowing your body to gradually return to normal cardiovascular function; stretching your warm muscles; and rehydrating. Cooling down doesn't require props and you can do it anywhere: on the trail, on the dock, or in your backyard.

First, slow your heart rate and breathing by continuing your activity at a slower rate—walking or swimming a couple of easy laps, for example—for five to ten minutes. Then, take advantage of the warmth of your muscles to stretch (combining stretching with regular exercise is the best way to prevent injury because your muscles become both stronger and more flexible in the process). Finally, remember that you have been sweating a lot while exercising—begin replacing your fluids as soon as you slow down. Drink water in small sips throughout your cooldown.

Your cooldown routine may be the best part of your workout—and you may decide to use the following stretches every day to stay limber and relaxed.

Stretches for Pregnancy

Stretching during pregnancy feels great and helps alleviate common aches and pains. It will also improve your flexibility for delivery. After activity—especially if you have broken a sweat—your muscles are most pliable and easiest to stretch. Remember, your goal during pregnancy is not to permanently lengthen your muscles but to release and relax them.

Be careful when stretching—you can do damage if you are not gentle. If any stretch hurts, stop. Keep in mind that your ligaments and joints become more vulnerable during pregnancy, so overstretching can easily strain a muscle or, worse, injure a joint.

Because of your growing uterus, your abdominal muscles can separate (called *diastasis recti*) during pregnancy—especially if you stretch them. It is safe to build your abdominal muscles but not a good idea to stretch them during pregnancy. Before exercising, run your finger along the *linea alba*, the vertical line between your belly button and pubic bone, to check for any separation of the abdominal muscles—this will heal after delivery. If you feel anything unusual, contact your doctor and avoid strenuous exercise and any movements that stretch the abdominal muscles.

Safe Stretching During Pregnancy

- **Avoid overstretching your muscles and joints—stop before it hurts.**

- **Avoid stretching your abdominal muscles.**

- **Avoid being upside down (with your head below your heart) while stretching.**

- **Avoid stretches that cramp or put pressure on your uterus (such as toe touches).**

- **Avoid lying on your back for long periods—stay upright or lie on your side.**

- **Avoid stretches (such as the hurdler's stretch) that strain your pelvic joints.**

Any stretches that require you to be upside down are not safe during pregnancy, since you may become light-headed if your head is below your heart. Also, avoid lying on your back for longer than a couple of minutes, particularly after twenty weeks, as the weight of your uterus can slow blood flow to your heart and to your fetus. You will have to modify your favorite stretching routine; the stretches described here are simple, safe, and comfortable, even in late pregnancy.

The best after-exercise stretches work the muscles that you just used and are still warm. A few stretches described here help relieve tension in your back and neck; use these throughout the day to relax. If you have an achy muscle—in your lower back, for example—use a stretch to gently relieve muscle strain and improve flexibility. Most outdoor exercises use many muscle groups, so I've designed the stretches below to be used after any workout—or even after a quick jaunt like taking the dog for a stroll.

Extend the muscle until you feel a stretch, but not to the point of pain. Hold each stretch at least ten to thirty seconds and keep breathing as the muscle relaxes. Stretch a little further and hold another ten to thirty seconds. Don't bounce: do a smooth, relaxed stretch for each muscle group.

Neck Stretches for Pregnancy

Side Neck Stretch. Tilt your head to the side, with your ear dropping toward your shoulder, then straighten and tilt your head the other way. Keep your shoulders down and relaxed. You should feel the stretch along the side of your neck into your shoulder. Repeat the side-to-side stretch ten times.

Forward Neck Circles. With your back straight, tilt your head forward to look down toward your belly. You'll feel the stretch in the back of your neck. Gently roll your head from side to side in half circles. Try ten half circles.

Shoulder Stretches for Pregnancy

Front Shoulder Stretch. While standing or sitting, reach your arms behind you with your palms facing each other and your elbows straight, and clasp your hands together behind your lower back. Raise your linked hands upward so that you feel the stretch in your shoulders, chest, and arms. Hold for ten to thirty seconds.

Back Shoulder Stretch. While standing or sitting, draw your straightened right arm across your chest and place your left hand just above the elbow to press your arm toward you, so that you feel the stretch in your right shoulder and upper arm. Hold for ten seconds and repeat on the other side.

Arm Stretches for Pregnancy

Side Stretch. Stand with your feet shoulder-width apart or sit. Reach one arm up toward the ceiling, keeping the other hand on a chair or on your hip for support. Look up toward your raised hand. You should feel the stretch along your arm and down the side of your body. Hold for a count of ten seconds and repeat on the other side.

Bent-Over Arm Stretch. Stand several feet behind a chair (or other sturdy surface) and bend forward at the hips until your upper body is parallel with the floor and your hands rest on the back of the chair. Your body should form a straight line from your hands to your buttocks. Gently press into your hands so that you feel the stretch in your arms and chest. Pull in your abdominal muscles to support the lower back and avoid arching. Hold for a count of ten seconds.

Triceps Stretch. Stand or sit with one arm bent behind your head with the hand resting in the middle of your back. Use the other hand to gently press your elbow so that you feel the stretch in your triceps. Hold for a count of ten seconds and repeat on the other side.

Back Stretches for Pregnancy

Back Curve Stretch. Sit on the floor with your knees bent in front of you. Hold the backs of your thighs with your hands and suck in your abdominals so that your back is rounded into a C shape. This stretches your lower back and buttocks. Hold for ten seconds, then release and straighten your spine.

Back Twist. Sit on the floor with your knees bent and your back straight. Twist to one side so that you are looking behind you and are using your opposite hand on your leg to pull yourself around. Hold for ten to thirty seconds, then release and face forward. Twist and stretch to the other side.

Pelvic Stretches for Pregnancy

Inner Thigh Stretch. Sit with the soles of your feet together so that your legs are open like a book. You'll feel the stretch in your inner thighs. Do not press down on your thighs, since the hip joint is vulnerable to injury during pregnancy. Stop if you feel strain in your groin. Stay in this position for ten to thirty seconds, release and straighten your legs, then repeat.

Squat Stretch. Stand with your feet a little more than shoulder-distance apart with your toes pointed out to the sides (if this hurts your knees, keep your toes pointed more forward). Keeping your back straight and your hips tucked under you, lower down into a squat as far as you can go, keeping your heels on the floor. Press the palms of your hands onto your inner thighs above the knees and gently push outward, so your pelvis opens. Feel the stretch through the inner thigh and groin. Hold for fifteen seconds, then stand. Repeat once. As you practice this, you'll be able to hold the squat for increasingly longer periods of time, which will really limber up your pelvis for delivery.

Hip Stretch. Stand with your left leg about one foot in front of your right. Raise your right heel off the floor so that the right knee is slightly bent. Gently tuck your buttocks under you and press the bottom of your hips forward so that you feel the stretch through the front of your thighs. Hold for ten seconds, then release and stand straight. Repeat on the other side.

Leg Stretches for Pregnancy

Hamstring Stretch. Stand with your right leg two feet in front of your left. Bend your left knee and place both hands on your right thigh. Flex the toes on your right foot and bend forward with a flat back to stretch the back of your right thigh. Hold for ten seconds, release and roll up to a standing position, and repeat on the other side.

Quadriceps Stretch. Stand with one hand on a sturdy surface for support. Bend your right knee, reach back with your right hand, and grab the ankle. Feel the stretch in the muscles in the front of your right thigh. Hold for ten to thirty seconds, release, and repeat on the other side.

Calf Stretch. Stand facing a wall (or tree). Place the toes of your right foot against the wall and flex, pointing them up as far as you can. Gently lean forward until you feel a stretch in your calf muscles. Hold for ten seconds and repeat on the other side.

Outer Thigh Stretch. Lie on your right side with your right leg extended straight. Bend your left leg and bring your left foot in front of your right leg, pulling your left knee toward your chest. You'll feel the stretch in your outer thigh and buttocks. Hold for ten seconds, release, turn over, and repeat on the other side.

If you are not very flexible, start slowly, and stop before the stretch becomes painful. As you stretch, focus on the muscles you are targeting; you are doing it right if that's where you feel the stretch. Stretching, alone or as part of an exercise routine, is a healthy way to care for your muscles, gently calm your body and mind after a good workout, and ready your body for childbirth.

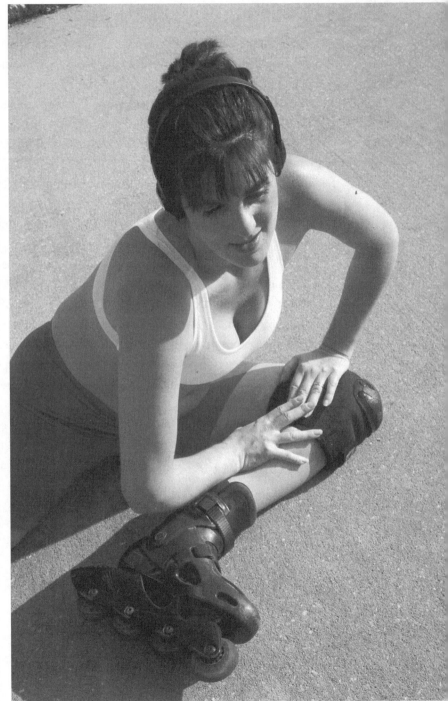

chapter 8

GARDENING

• • •

WALKING

• • •

RUNNING

• • •

BIKING

• • •

IN-LINE SKATING

Staying Active near Home

Staying active during pregnancy does not mean you have to be a rough-and-tumble outdoorswoman or scale glaciers in your free time. Most of the activities we love and enjoy often can be done close to home and include the great outdoors just out the front door.

Walking the dog, raking leaves, and biking through the local park are the day-to-day behaviors that define us as active women. Until you're pregnant, you may not even consider what good exercise some of these activities can be. During pregnancy, these close-to-home excursions may become a healthy part of your routine.

Convenience is part of what makes these nearby activities so attractive during pregnancy. You can always just turn around and head home. And you can stick close to your phone and family. It's easy to squeeze a little gardening time or a quick jog into an otherwise demanding schedule—and you can take as much or as little time as you've got handy.

If you run, skate, garden, bike, or walk regularly, doing these activities will now feel different to you, and you'll have to alter your routine, especially as the pregnancy progresses. Your posture will change, your stance will widen, your joints will relax, your uterus will get in the way, and your stamina will, let's face it, diminish. Before you know it, you'll have to adjust according to the time, intensity, and distance you feel comfortable with. But as pregnancy enriches your life, you'll find that these near-home excursions are excellent preparation for an active motherhood.

gardening

Growing your own fresh vegetables is deeply satisfying, second only to growing your own baby. Nurturing seedlings from sprouts to flowers to fruits puts you intimately in touch with the natural process. By cultivating a garden, you create a beautiful, evolving world around you—one that attracts birds and bees. The garden also invites you to spend long hours in its shade, caring for it and enjoying its color. During pregnancy, many women feel like gardening because their "nesting" instincts have kicked in and they want to make their home as cozy as possible before the baby arrives. Or maybe they've always enjoyed gardening as a way to spend time outdoors and get their hands dirty.

Gardening is also about healthy eating. The big benefit of organic gardening—which is especially important during pregnancy—is being able to avoid the pesticides, insecticides, radiation, genetic engineering, waxes, and preservatives used on market fruits and vegetables. Healthy eating is good for you in the long run, but feasting on fresh-picked fruits and vegetables, homegrown or store bought, during pregnancy will also give you some immediate nutritional benefits. For example, during your first trimester, when fatigue and morning sickness are making you feel lousy, a balanced meal with plenty of vegetables will help you get the nutrients you need—and maybe even make you feel less nauseous and more energetic. When your nausea subsides between meals or you just need more food, fruits are an excellent snack and the natural sugars will boost your energy without filling you up with lots of empty calories. Take a look at the chart on page 88 of some of the nutritional demands of pregnancy and the fruits and veggies that help meet those needs.

Even a balanced diet may not meet all of your needs, so keep taking that daily prenatal vitamin and any supplements your doctor recommends (like iron). Eating plenty of fruits and vegetables will just make it easier for your body to absorb and use those nutrients. The fresher the produce and the more vibrant the color, the more nutrients you're getting with each bite—that's why homegrown veggies are so good for you.

But what about the *work* of gardening? Gardening is one of the few activities you can enjoy right up to your delivery date—and get right back to afterward, during those short hours when your newborn naps (just bring that baby monitor outside with you). Playing with dirt is fundamentally relaxing and, if you're new to gardening, you'll find that you enjoy it as much as your youngster soon will.

Gardening is good exercise, especially later in pregnancy when simply walking around the garden and squatting to pull weeds will get your heart pumping. Raking, pruning, digging, planting, mulching, mowing, and weeding give you a good workout without even seeming like exercise. I guarantee you'll be sweating. As you reach up to pick apples off the tree, you're stretching your arms and back. Carrying baskets of fruit, you're strengthening those muscles too. Raking works your upper body, and squatting to pull weeds works your lower body. Plus, gardening is a convenient form of exercise, since you don't need to go anywhere, you don't need special equipment, and the garden *always* needs more work.

RISK ASSESSMENT BY TRIMESTER

1ST TRIMESTER: LOW
2ND TRIMESTER: LOW
3RD TRIMESTER: LOW

Staying Healthy Each Trimester

1ST TRIMESTER | RISK: LOW

Gardening is a very safe and healthy activity throughout pregnancy. As long as you keep your balance around the rose bushes and don't disturb a wasp's nest, you are not likely to hurt yourself. During your first trimester, you may just not feel up for big outdoor excursions, and taking care of your garden is a great way to get outdoors without having to change out of your pajamas and flip-flops. Plus, putting delicious fresh veggies from your own garden on your table will help you have a healthier diet and curb your unhealthy cravings.

During your first trimester, try to get out in the garden for ten to fifteen minutes every day, whether you are picking off deadheads, trimming herbs, or simply watering. Make time two or three times a week for larger garden projects, like planting, mowing, weeding, pruning, or mulching. Any passionate gardener knows that a garden thrives with regular attention. You'll notice the difference in your plants and in your own peace of mind.

When you're out in your garden, make sure you protect your delicate skin from sunburn and stay cool. A big hat helps. Even if you're just replanting flowers, take breaks in the shade and keep yourself well hydrated. Keep a big jug of water—or lemonade—nearby.

gardening

Now that your belly is bigger, you have a few more comfort and safety issues to consider, even when gardening in your own backyard. The shift in your posture will affect how you stand, squat, and work outside. As your weight increases, you'll need more leg strength to change position and crouching may become uncomfortable—or difficult to get up from. Try sitting on a low stool when working on the ground. While you are sitting, hold your back upright, not hunched, and keep your weight balanced on your sitting bones. This trimester, you'll still be able to work around your belly pretty effectively.

Since your fetus is obviously growing out of your pelvis, where it was well protected, your balance may be impaired. Avoid climbing ladders and trees and watch your step on uneven ground.

Your back is doing the difficult work of supporting your growing belly, so it is also more vulnerable to soreness and the aching that will keep you out of the garden. Protect your back by avoiding heavy lifting; get help when moving the wheelbarrow or dumping a bag of potting soil. If you must lift something—a potted plant or a tray of seedlings—lift slowly; keep your legs well apart and stable, bending at the knees and lifting with your arms and legs, rather than with your back. And get up and stretch—often.

If you've always done a bit of gardening, you'll enjoy the peace and quiet of getting out this trimester and you'll be able to keep your garden in great shape without making a lot of adjustments. Aim for fifteen minutes of garden time a day. It doesn't sound like a lot, but you can make a lot of progress in a quarter of an hour, whether you are sweeping the deck, trimming hedges, securing climbers, or repotting.

Set aside two hours a week for more involved garden projects, like intensive work on one part of the garden. Use this time to make your yard into a child-friendly environment. Are the cacti out of reach? Is the pond gracefully fenced off? Have you worked in lawn or patio space to accommodate a playpen, a swing, or even a sandbox? If you haven't been very active so far this pregnancy, gardening is a terrific way to get out of the house, improve your yard, get in good shape for your third trimester—and get a chance to *eat* the fruits of your labor.

"

Getting outdoors allowed me to preserve my identity as an active woman who was about to become a mother. There is so much anticipation when you're pregnant, so something to pass the time is always welcome. And I didn't have the energy to plan outings. So, I did a lot of gardening.

I was a little afraid that it would be a long time before I could get outside again after the baby was born—which turned out to be true. Being in the garden is the exception, though—we're out there every day.

I gardened less for physical exercise than as a form of spiritual meditation. Being pregnant is the ultimate excuse for accepting and taking care of your body. For the first time, maybe ever, I didn't care what I looked like, at least most of the time. I wore anything that would fit and I felt good. People would smile at me, start conversations, and generally look kindly upon me everywhere I went. The hard part was realizing, after the baby was born, that I couldn't immediately go back to the old clothes that I had anticipated would fit again. But it felt good to take that break from my usual hectic, high-energy lifestyle.

We joke about nesting behaviors during pregnancy, and the garden really was my nest. It was gorgeous! During my eighth and ninth months, I was out there all the time because gardening made me feel productive and fulfilled. I could also be close to the phone and the car. Truthfully, gardening was tiring and I would get flushed and need lots of naps. I found it easy to get outside to work in the garden, though, and it felt like the very least I could do and still be somewhat active.

—Tracy, Memphis, Tennessee

"

gardening

PREGNANCY MEANS:	THE NUTRIENT YOU NEED	NATURAL SOURCE
Acne	Vitamin B_6	Bananas, dried fruit, greens
Anemia	Iron	Beans, nuts, spinach
Constipation	Fiber	Apples, apricots, plums
Fatigue	Vitamin B_1	Peas, nuts, sunflower seeds
Fetus's bone and organ growth	Vitamin A	Fruits, greens, yellow peppers
Fetus's bone and teeth growth	Phosphorus	Fruits, vegetables
Fetus's brain and spinal cord development	Folic acid (folate)	Asparagus, beans, dark green leafy vegetables, fruit
Fetus's growth and development	Vitamin B_1 (thiamin)	Peas, nuts, sunflower seeds
Insulin and sugar regulation	Chromium	Bananas, mushrooms
Insulin and sugar regulations	Zinc	Beans, legumes
Mom and fetus's bone and muscle development	Magnesium	Beans, dark green leafy vegetables, fruits, nuts
Mom and fetus's bone growth	Vitamin D	Sunshine
Mood swings	Vitamin B_6	Bananas, dried fruit, greens
Morning sickness	Vitamin B_6	Bananas, dried fruit, greens
Stress	Pantothenic acid	Beans, green leafy vegetables
Varicose veins and increased blood volume	Vitamin C	Berries, cauliflower, dark green vegetables, melons, potatoes, yellow and red bell peppers
Vomiting	Potassium	Bananas, green leafy vegetables, legumes, mushrooms, oranges, yams

3RD TRIMESTER | RISK: LOW

This is when your gardening will really feel good—during this trimester when most other outdoor activities seem like a chore. Gardening fulfills your emotional need to prepare your home for the baby and allows you to stay near the house and phone while soaking in some sunshine. Gardening also gives you an incredible feeling of productivity during those last months when you start to feel like an immobile incubator.

Get a pair of clippers and trim some bushes, do a little light raking, and water the plants you worked hard on last trimester. It's time for maintenance work. Stick to activities at waist level or above, like working at a garden table to replant seedlings into pots, snipping buds, or cutting back hedges. Also, avoid bending over to work on the ground—you could become dizzy and fall.

If you're still limber enough to sit on a low stool, you can do some weeding, but I recommend delegating ground activities as your pregnancy progresses. If you're standing while gardening, try putting one foot on a brick or footstool with your knee bent to prevent strain on your lower back. Even when mowing or raking, keep your back straight and your hips tucked under you, so that your belly isn't thrust forward, avoiding that deep arch in your lower back—the rules of good posture hold, whether you're watering fruit trees or sitting on the deck admiring your day's work.

You'll notice right away that you're getting a good workout. Even a few trips around the garden to check out the latest ripe veggies and newly opened roses will do the trick. Cut down on your time in the sun, since you are particularly vulnerable to dehydration late in pregnancy. Plan your outside time for the morning or evening when the garden is cool. You can keep up the ten-minute a day routine, but limit larger projects to half an hour at a time, so that you get hydrated and off your feet regularly. At this pace, you can keep up with your garden right up to delivery.

gardening

Equipment Considerations

You won't need any new equipment to garden during pregnancy—I promise the old clippers and shovels will still work fine. But I recommend that you pull a few things out of the shed to make gardening more comfortable—and safer. Dirt can transmit bacterial infections. Plus, exposure to fertilizers and pesticides can be dangerous—even if you have only brief contact with recently sprayed plants. However, simply wearing gloves when gardening and composting will protect you well. Find a pair made of thick canvas with a rubber or suede exterior surface to protect you from rose thorn punctures or scratches from straw or wood splinters, which can expose you to fungal infections. Likewise, don't handle any animal scat—even your own kitty's—while working outside. As good as the fertile earth feels to your bare feet, wearing socks and shoes is a good idea to avoid fungal infections on your feet and legs. When you're done gardening for the day, wash your hands thoroughly with mild soap and warm water, scrubbing out any dirt lodged under your fingernails with a nail brush.

If it is very dry outside—especially in parts of the western United States where desert winds can whip up a lot of dust—wet down the area you will be working on with a light spray of water, so that you don't breath a lot of dust while working.

If you're working in an uncultivated area where there may be poison oak or ivy or other rough bushes, like blackberry, wear long sleeves and long pants. You may have a more severe skin reaction to irritating plants during pregnancy— that means lots of itching and redness, which you'll have to treat with cool, moist towels and a lot of patience.

Instead of kneeling or crouching on the ground when gardening, try using a low stool that is wide enough to comfortably sit on and six to twelve inches off the ground. Until later in your third trimester, when settling down onto it will become a challenge in itself, a low seat is a great way to protect your back and legs, keep your back straighter, stretch your legs to maintain healthy blood flow and prevent varicose veins, and put less pressure on your delicate joints.

Planning Pointers for Pregnancy

1 Garden for today and tomorrow. When you garden, you reap the immediate rewards of staying active: having more energy, maintaining your stamina and flexibility, and enjoying a positive outlook. But the benefits keep on coming. An apricot tree you plant now will be a cherished reminder of your pregnancy for years to come—it becomes a part of your child's history. An apricot from your own garden is an appetizing healthy snack that helps to combat constipation. Plus, those nutritious and tasty fruits and vegetables—which are pesticide, fertilizer, and insecticide free—will become a healthy part of your family's diet.

2 Use a stool. Save your back and make it easier to get up and down by sitting on a low stool while weeding and replanting. Using a stool will also maintain good circulation to your legs and help prevent varicose veins, spider veins, and leg and ankle swelling.

3 Wear gloves. Protect your hands from punctures, scratches, contact with irritating plants, and possible bacteria in the dirt. And wash your hands and scrub under your fingernails when you're done in the garden.

4 Make yourself comfortable. The garden is such a tempting place that you'll want to be out there a while. So put on something comfortable, set aside a pair of dirty, supportive shoes (try some gardening clogs that can be hosed down when they get too caked in mud), and keep a wide-brimmed hat handy. You may even decide to designate a firm cushion and a supportive chair as garden gear and take them out with you.

gardening

5   Take a breather. Gardening is good exercise, but it's easy to get carried away. You may only be twenty steps from your kitchen but forget to refuel. Make sure you are taking breaks, drinking plenty of water, and eating snacks before you get too worn out.

6   Watch the sun. An afternoon of ardent gardening, even on cloudy days, can leave you sunburned and dehydrated if you aren't careful. Put on that sunscreen, stick to the shade during the sunniest times of the day (noon to four in the afternoon), wear a big hat, and set up an outdoor umbrella—it will protect you while you work and look great in the garden.

7   Avoid the heat. Avoid gardening on very hot or humid days, when you may overheat: you'll feel lousy and it's not good for your fetus. Your garden will still be right there in a couple of hours or days when it has cooled off.

8   Have a vision. Maintaining a clear idea of what you hope to do with your garden in the next few months (for example, "put in a colorful flower border along the driveway") will give you the satisfaction of working toward and accomplishing your goals. When it feels like you've been pregnant forever, those blossoms will remind you that you—and your fetus—have made some good progress.

walking

Walking is a great way to stay in shape during pregnancy without a lot of fuss. Whether you're fit or you've never exercised before, you can enjoy—and benefit from—taking a walk. Staying fit shouldn't be a chore and walking may be the one exercise that really fits in your plans and doesn't wear you out. If you're really busy, you've always enjoyed walking, or if you're just starting to get used to a more active lifestyle, walking is a good choice.

And it's good exercise. Walking will get your heart pumping, especially during pregnancy. And it will work out your entire body and firm up your muscles. Walking is an aerobic exercise, so it revs up your heart and lungs and builds your stamina. You'll thank yourself during labor, when you need that extra endurance. Walking is also a weight-bearing exercise, which means that simply carrying your weight helps strengthen your bones and gives you a good workout, but it also doesn't strain your joints the way running or hiking might.

You can make walking a part of your routine in many little ways. No matter where you live, you're only a few steps from the great outdoors. Look out for neighborhood trails, bike paths, city parks, and even scenic shaded streets as good walking destinations. Use lunch breaks to walk a few laps around a nearby park or stroll to the deli. And yes, it counts if you walk around inside the mall if it's just too hot, cold, or rainy outside. It even counts when you park at the far end of the parking lot and walk to the store or when you take your dog for a stroll around the neighborhood.

Walking is a low-risk activity during pregnancy. This means that it's healthy for you and your baby and it won't endanger your pregnancy, as long as you give your body the extra attention it needs when you do any form of exercise: drink lots of water and take frequent breaks. If you feel too worn out, just stop and try again another day.

Ideally, you'll gradually increase your walking routine so that you are walking three to six days a week. You'll notice the benefits: you'll have less back and pelvic pain, you'll have more energy, and you'll be more relaxed. Walking is better preparation for labor and delivery than swimming, since it is a weight-bearing exercise and may result in a shorter labor and fewer complications and interventions at birth. Walking is also a healthy habit you'll want to keep up after delivery— and your baby will really enjoy going out with you too.

walking

RISK ASSESSMENT BY TRIMESTER

> **1ST TRIMESTER: LOW**
> **2ND TRIMESTER: LOW**
> **3RD TRIMESTER: LOW**

Staying Healthy Each Trimester

1ST TRIMESTER | RISK: LOW

You'll find it pretty easy to make walking a part of your day, even in early pregnancy when you may feel sick and exhausted. After all, all you need is a pair of shoes and enough motivation to get out the door. That's not to say that walking won't wear you out. Your pregnancy demands a lot from your body, especially during these first months, so you'll get tired quickly; that's normal. Just walk as far as you can, as often as you can.

Walking will get easier as you get in shape and get used to the pregnancy—and it will also make your pregnancy easier down the road. The fresh air may help with nausea and the regular exercise may reduce insomnia.

As your fetus is developing its vital organs, you should be careful to stay cool. Don't walk on hot or humid days or in areas where there is no shade, in case you get hot and need a break. In order to stay hydrated, always carry a water bottle on a walk longer than twenty minutes.

If it's too hot to be outside, try a stroll through a big air-conditioned store—the scenery won't be as good, but you'll get some exercise if you don't stop to shop. If you're headed out on a warm day, wear light layers and peel them off as you heat up (but keep your skin covered so you don't burn) and walk during cooler times of the day.

If you're new to exercise and are just starting out, try walking on a flat path for five to ten minutes every day. It doesn't sound like a lot, but your workout should also include a five-minute warm-up (try some dynamic stretching; see chapter 6) and a five-minute cooldown. Add a few minutes to the routine every week until you are regularly walking for one-half hour at least three times a week.

The more you walk, the stronger your heart and lungs become and the better they will be able to support your fetus later in pregnancy. If you can get in the habit of walking now, you'll have an easier time staying active later in pregnancy.

"I've never been a particularly athletic woman and, during my pregnancy, I have reveled in the fact that I don't have to exercise if I don't want to. But I live in downtown San Francisco, where the parking is scarce and the people watching is excellent, and you just can't do anything without also doing some walking.

So, most of my walking is in town—on streets and in parks. I always wear comfortable shoes and avoid the killer hills. During pregnancy, I haven't changed my habits much. With all the new feelings I was having during the first trimester, I wasn't ready to take on more challenging activities.

I have even started borrowing a friend's dog just to get out of the house. At this point, I've got my favorite walking routines down. It's a perfect ten-minute walk to Dolores Park: full of sunshine and little kids on the swings. And it's a fifteen-minute walk to 24th Street, teeming with street vendors and good window-shopping. Both places are very tempting destinations and they don't tend to take too much out of me.

The funny thing is that since my fifth month people have noticed that I am waddling. I even amuse myself with my "ducky" posture. In the last two months, I've really started to slow down. What was a fifteen-minute walk to and from my watercolor class has turned into a twenty-five minute trudge.

I'm a few weeks from my due date and I'm huge and sore—more sore than most pregnant women I know, it seems. If I walk for twenty minutes, I get home and have to lose my shoes immediately and put my feet up. But I also feel that walking improves my posture—and the exercise certainly helps me sleep better. Even an amble through the park feels like terrific exercise.

—Jen, San Francisco, California"

walking

2ND TRIMESTER | RISK: LOW

The second trimester is a good time to get back in shape or increase your fitness level, since you'll have more energy and will feel like getting out and about. Walking is a good solution.

If you don't feel up for anything more active, you may want to just take an evening stroll near home to get some fresh air. You shouldn't have difficulty walking the same routes you enjoyed before pregnancy; paved paths are easiest. If you're just starting out, take it easy on the hills and make the walk fun so that you stay motivated. Your fetus will enjoy it too, since evidence points to the fact that babies can feel your rhythmic steps from inside the uterus.

If you've been exercising all along and want a little challenge, choose paths with some hills, if you can, so that you enhance your cardiovascular workout. Find a park with some gently sloping paths or just pace yourself to maximize your workout: after warming up for five minutes, walk for six, speed walk for six to get your heart pumping, and then stroll for six before cooling down and stretching out those muscles.

You'll probably have enough stamina, especially after your sixth month, to combine walking with other activities like biking to get an even better aerobic workout.

3RD TRIMESTER | RISK: LOW

The great advantage to walking is that you can keep it up during your third trimester, right up to your delivery. Your belly may really throw you off balance if you try hiking, biking, or swimming at this point, but it's an advantage when it comes to walking. It'll give you a better workout in less time, since carrying that extra weight will work your heart, lungs, and muscles more rigorously.

You may not need to change your routine much if you're already walking local groomed paths. Your chances of tripping and falling are pretty slim if you're on a sidewalk. You will get out of breath quickly, however, even on flat paths, so take breaks and head home before you feel worn out. Many women also experience low pelvic pain—a brief, sharp jolt—with walking, as the round ligaments that support the uterus get stretched; this pain resolves with rest. Your big belly also puts pressure on your diaphragm, making it difficult for you to take a deep breath. And your belly puts a lot of strain on your back muscles, so walking may tire your back out—although, in the long run, regular exercise will help strengthen those muscles. Regardless, the change of scenery and quiet time spent outdoors will feel really good, even if you're just walking around the block.

As with any aerobic exercise, if you're working hard, you may notice some intermittent tightening across your belly while walking toward the end of your pregnancy. These Braxton Hicks contractions are common and they should go away if you stop and rest for a few minutes.

This trimester, walking is an excellent way to get outdoors. Neighborhood parks offer safe, flat paths that won't challenge your balance or take you too far from home. Even if you've been exercising throughout this pregnancy, set modest goals and ramp down your routine as your body sends signals of fatigue: sweating, breathlessness, and achiness.

Break down your half-hour routine into ten minutes of warming up, ten of walking at a comfortable pace, and ten of cooling down and hydrating. You can incorporate some breathing exercises into your warm-up. Learning to coordinate your breathing with using your muscles and stretching is great preparation for labor. The pace of walking allows you to focus on your breathing, using the pressure on your diaphragm from the uterus to help you breathe out fully before inhaling. Don't try to slow your breathing while exercising, however, since you will naturally have a faster respiratory rate in pregnancy.

As you get close to your due date and especially if you pass your due date, your doctor may encourage you to walk as much as you can—it makes the baby happy and may stimulate the start of labor. Even during labor, walking around can help the contractions become more regular and effective and speed up your cervical dilation.

Warming Up

Start walking slowly with an easy stride on flat ground for two to three minutes. Then do some dynamic stretches to activate the muscles you rely on when walking: focus on your legs, back, and hips (see chapter 6). Warm up thoroughly before walking briskly or heading uphill will help you prevent injuries and soreness.

walking

Walking Technique for Pregnancy

Posture is especially important when walking. Poor posture strains your muscles and joints and leaves you tired and sore—and unwilling to continue walking. If you can develop a good posture when walking, you'll manage to stand and sit straighter too.

Pregnancy affects your posture by bringing your center of gravity forward so that you are inclined to arch your back. Check your posture in front of a mirror. Looking at your body in profile, your shoulders should line up with your hips so that your lower back is not drastically curved. Use your stomach muscles to tuck your pelvis under a little—this will help align your spine and may protect you from injuring your back.

Keep your back in line by holding your head and chest up; watching the ground will give you a sore back. Swing your arms when you walk and bend your arms at the elbow so that they are propelling you forward at a ninety-degree angle. You may notice that you have a tendency to bend forward at the waist when you want to walk faster or are heading uphill. Instead, lean your entire body a little bit forward to give yourself some momentum while keeping your back straight.

You are walking at a healthy pace if you are breathing hard but can still talk comfortably. Break a sweat and get your heart pumping. But if you get too hot or short of breath, slow down for a bit, then keep walking.

Cooling Down

As you near the end of your walk, slow down your pace for a couple of minutes to allow your heart rate to return to normal. Then take a few minutes to stretch while your muscles are warm, to increase your flexibility and prevent soreness. Pay particular attention to stretching the muscles in your legs: the hamstrings, quadriceps, and your calves. If you're heading back to your workplace, take advantage of these few minutes to stretch your shoulders and back, which can get tense during the day. If you find that your ankles become swollen after walking, sit down and elevate your feet after you cool down, to get that extra blood to circulate back to your heart.

Equipment Considerations

What makes walking such a convenient exercise is the fact that all you need are some good shoes. If you've found some supportive shoes with a flat sole that you're comfortable in all day during pregnancy, they'll probably work for walking. Uncomfortable shoes can give you blisters and make back pain worse. If you're going on long walks or walking hills, look into getting some athletic shoes. Besides shoes, consider wearing a hat for sun protection and a small backpack to carry your water. If you're walking at night or in an area with bicycle or car traffic, take the usual precautions and think about wearing a reflective vest or jacket so you are very visible.

Preparing for Difficult Situations

When choosing a walking path, get a sense of the inclines and total distance before heading out, and make sure you have adequate shoes, shade, and water. Walking on pavement is important too; traversing a gravel or uneven path is risky if you are not wearing closed and supportive walking shoes or if you can't visualize each step. If you're heading out on your own, check for cell phone access, and don't forget to look out for benches, restrooms, and park service patrols, just in case you need them.

If you're going to be walking in an urban area, your risks don't change a whole lot now that you are pregnant. You'll still be watching for traffic and sticking to safe, well-populated routes. Try to stay away from very busy roads where you'd be inhaling a lot of exhaust—there is no proof that those fumes are harmful, but common sense tells us that they can't be healthy. And, whether you're headed around the block or along a coastal walking path, keep an eye on the weather and tie an extra sweatshirt around your waist if necessary.

BASALT REGIONAL LIBRARY
99 MIDLAND AVENUE
BASALT CO 81621-8305

Planning Pointers for Pregnancy

1 Plan a shorter walk; walk more often. Walk shorter distances more frequently so that you stay motivated and build your stamina. Aim to walk an energizing half hour several times a week rather than an exhausting two-hour walk once a week. Work up to a regular schedule of walking for at least half an hour (that may mean a half mile or two miles, depending on how fast you walk) three to six times a week.

2 Adjust your equipment. Always walk in your most comfortable shoes. Footwear with good arch and ankle support is key during pregnancy—especially if you are walking on hills or uneven surfaces. Carry water in a backpack, even for a short walk.

3 Take a friend. You'll enjoy your walk more and be safer in case of a problem if you're with someone.

4 Avoid the heat. Avoid walking outside on hot or humid days. Always choose routes with shade and take frequent breaks, especially if you are heading uphill.

5 Warm up and cool down. Even if you're not sweating a lot, you are giving your body a good workout and you'll need to take a few minutes to warm up, cool down, and stretch to prevent injuries and soreness and to build stamina and flexibility. Don't skip it!

6 Know how to get help. Bring a cell phone or at least some change for a pay phone in case you need help. Stay in well-traveled areas during your third trimester.

7 Have fun. Walking is a great way to enjoy a friend's company, get away from your daily stress, and take time for yourself while conditioning your body and preparing yourself and your fetus for a healthy delivery.

running

If you were a committed runner or jogger before getting pregnant, you can continue to enjoy your routine, though slightly modified, during pregnancy. If you are fit, running is healthy for you and your baby. You are probably in very good shape—you have to be if you're a runner—and most exercise will be easier for you during pregnancy. This means that you can keep running or jogging with an eye on avoiding overexertion and joint strain. Don't be surprised if you can't run as far or as fast as you used to; your heart is working for two—a workout in itself. Be flexible about how you define a "run": it is okay and healthy to slow your pace, skip the sprinting, and throw in some walking along the way. In my mind, running, jogging, and brisk walking all count as a run, since you will get a good workout doing any of the three.

Running is a low-risk exercise during pregnancy if you are fit. I don't recommend starting a running program during pregnancy because it can strain your muscles and joints—especially with that extra weight—and your heart if you are not already in good cardiovascular shape.

Like walking, running is a *weight-bearing* exercise, meaning that simply carrying your own weight makes the action more strenuous and builds both your muscles and bones. Since you start panting within minutes of starting a run, you know that running is also excellent *aerobic* exercise, helping to make your heart and lungs stronger and more efficient. You can probably imagine how that regular deep breathing while jogging will help you breathe through labor and keep your stamina up for pushing during delivery.

Running is one of the best-studied exercises during pregnancy. And the results of all those studies are positive: regular running (or jogging)—at least three times a week—will prepare you well for the rigors of labor and will prevent aches, fatigue, nausea, high blood sugar, and leg cramps during pregnancy. You'll have less stress, more energy, and a better attitude. Plus, you are more likely to have a less painful and shorter labor and a more responsive and maybe even a more intelligent baby. Rest assured that running doesn't cause miscarriages or preterm labor. You may find that the bouncing is a little uncomfortable for you, but it doesn't bother your baby a bit and the rhythmic movement provides him or her with healthy stimulation.

Many people begin running for its health benefits. Running is one of the quickest ways to burn calories and build endurance. But those shouldn't be the reasons you run during pregnancy. First, you want to *gain* weight during pregnancy and you should not use running to lose pounds at this time. Second, pregnancy is not a good time to train competitively. If you choose to run, do it to maintain your fitness level, not to increase it.

There are famous women runners who have competed in marathons during pregnancy and immediately afterward. Sure, it is possible, but I don't recommend it. Stay away from sprinting and racing. You don't want your exercise to take away from your fetus's growth and development. Plus, you don't want to exercise so intensely that you become exhausted, miserable, or worse, get injured. If you pace yourself and listen to your body, jogging (or run-walking) can be a very healthy part of your pregnancy and can make you feel energized, confident, and fit.

If you have always enjoyed running, you'll probably want to continue running during pregnancy. For some women, the challenge may be taking it easy and giving yourself a break. Your goals should be to get outside, break a sweat, and blow off some steam. Think about it this way: even a workout of brisk walking three times a week will prepare you well for your next marathon—labor.

RISK ASSESSMENT BY TRIMESTER

1ST TRIMESTER: LOW

2ND TRIMESTER: LOW

3RD TRIMESTER: MEDIUM

Staying Healthy Each Trimester

1ST TRIMESTER | RISK: LOW

If you feel up for running or jogging during your first trimester, go for it. You are lucky if running is already a part of your schedule and something you look forward to—it will be easier for you to stay motivated. Admittedly, you may just not feel like running much this trimester as your body makes some big adjustments to supporting your fetus. You can still stay in shape if you get out for brief jogs or run-walks. Bringing along your dog or choosing a favorite path may help keep your spirits up too. The more you are able to stay active this trimester, the better you'll feel and the easier it will be to continue exercising later in pregnancy.

Your priority this trimester is to learn to focus on your body—rather than your usual fitness goals. It is very important that you stay cool since your fetus's organs are developing and can be affected by overheating. This may mean cutting back your running time or avoiding big hills and sticking to level paths. Simply don't go running at all if it is too hot or humid—try an indoor treadmill instead. Peel off layers as you warm up, even in cool weather, but keep a layer on to protect your sensitive pregnancy skin from sunburn.

A healthy program involves both running and walking so that you get a good workout but avoid getting too hot or worn out. Always start by walking for five minutes to warm up. Then try running (or run-walking) for twelve minutes. Slow to a brisk walk for three minutes, then to a regular walk for another five minutes to cool down. If you are short on time, cut down on the running, but don't skip the warm-up and cooldown.

2ND TRIMESTER | RISK: LOW

During this trimester you'll probably have more energy and feel better able to run regularly—but don't push yourself. Stick with a routine that feels comfortable, rather than trying to meet competitive goals.

Running and jogging are tough on your muscles and joints, especially later in pregnancy. Even a quick jog may be uncomfortable for your lower back and belly because of the bouncing and stretching of the round ligaments that support your uterus. Wearing an abdominal girdle, a maternity belt, or even supportive bike shorts may help prevent this discomfort.

You may start to feel clumsy this trimester, tripping over your own feet or twisting an ankle as you hop off a curb. This clumsiness is to be expected as your body grows quickly, your center of gravity changes drastically, and your ligaments continue to relax. Watch your step and stick to flat, paved paths. Choose obstacle-free paths so that you can direct your attention inward. As you warm up, focus on your posture and arm swing. Notice that your feet strike the ground at a slightly different angle now. Your hips may also feel different as you walk—you may notice a bit of a waddling gait. Take time this trimester to get in touch with these subtle changes so that you are aware of your body and can learn to move safely and with confidence.

As an obstetrician, I am asked quite a few questions about exercise and pregnancy. I've concluded that it's really difficult for athletic high achievers to slow down during pregnancy. Especially psychologically. We are used to being active all the time.

I admit it: I'm an athletic high achiever too. So naturally I've been active this pregnancy—I can't imagine being otherwise. I've surfed. I've skied. I've biked. I've gardened. And I've managed to keep jogging almost to the end.

My pace has been slower and I'm more breathless, but I manage to cover the same distance as I did before pregnancy. I haven't had to change my gear. And I still devote myself to serious stretching with every workout.

At about twenty weeks, I developed some unnerving lower back pain, first on the right side, then on the left. Occasionally I had some pelvic pressure after exercise, and then, after twenty-nine weeks, while jogging. But stretching and continuing my exercise routine helped, I think.

At thirty-two weeks, my doctor became worried about preterm labor and asked me to stop all "unnecessary activities." That meant no running. And no stairs. I don't remember the last time I didn't exercise for three weeks. I didn't feel like myself. It was very hard.

By thirty-five weeks, the danger had passed—it would be safe to go into labor—and I started up again, taking to the trails for extended walks. And I'm still doing it at thirty-six weeks and five days!

—Kati, Denver, Colorado

running

If you've been running regularly, continue to ramp up your routine gently by alternating running and run-walking. When run-walking, tuck in your hips, straighten your spine, keep your elbows at right angles, and propel yourself forward using your whole body, including the swinging motion of your arms. This energetic walking will work all your muscles and improve your posture. Try walking for five minutes to warm up, running for ten, run-walking for five, running for another ten minutes, then run-walking for five before cooling down for five minutes. That's a total workout of forty minutes!

3RD TRIMESTER | RISK: MEDIUM

Even committed runners have trouble keeping up their enthusiasm during the third trimester because of the abdominal and joint strain resulting from carrying that heavy fetus and uterus and those extra fluids. The very weight of your pregnancy ensures an excellent workout just by walking briskly this trimester. It is easier than you think to stay in shape and you'll maintain your stamina, improve your sleep, stay fit for labor, and bounce back quickly after delivery.

You will be surprised to find that you are huffing and puffing even after your warm-up. This isn't because you've somehow become out of shape even after all that hard work to stay fit. What's happened is that your uterus has grown to over a thousand times its pre-pregnancy size and is putting a lot of pressure on your diaphragm (the muscle under your lungs), making it harder for you to catch your breath. Don't let feeling winded stop you from exercising— just slow down a bit. Staying fit will help your breathing be more efficient overall and may help prevent you from feeling short of breath during your daily activities, like climbing stairs or doing laundry. Also, if you exercise hard enough, your uterus will respond by tightening, or contracting. Rest for a few minutes and these Braxton Hicks contractions will go away.

Your goals this trimester are to get out of the house or office, do something active, and unwind, not to stay trim or build endurance. Use your workout time to appreciate how your baby responds to your activity (some babies kick a lot and some just lie back and enjoy the rocking) and to take a break from your responsibilities. If you can keep it up, you'll notice how good brisk walking makes you feel about your body.

As your pregnancy progresses this trimester, spend more time run-walking and less time running until you are walking briskly for a total of thirty minutes—plus ten minutes for warming up and cooling down. Even though you are running less, you'll still get an excellent workout since you are already working hard carrying the extra weight of your pregnancy. You'll maintain your aerobic fitness even though you are going slower and covering less ground. Aim to get your heart rate up for half an hour rather than covering a specific distance. Remember, the best workout is one you feel comfortable with and one that keeps you motivated.

Warming Up

Start walking slowly with an easy stride on flat ground for five minutes. Then do some dynamic stretches to activate the muscles you rely on when running, jogging, or brisk walking: focus on your legs, back, and hips (see chapter 6). Remember that being well warmed up will help you prevent injuries and soreness.

Running Technique for Pregnancy

You may feel that you mastered running around the time you learned to ride a tricycle and discarded your pacifier. But running, and even brisk walking, during pregnancy present a whole new challenge. Posture is especially important. Carrying that extra weight and compensating for relaxed ligaments mean that you have to pay attention to how you run. Carry your arms bent at a right angle at the level of your waist, hold your chin up, keep your shoulders and hips in line, and stay light on your feet.

If you ignore your posture, you'll find that your spine bends into an S shape with your lower back severely arched and your hips tipped forward. Plus, your feet will hit the pavement flat and turned out, like a duck's. Your muscles and joints will be strained and you'll have severe back pain. So before you head out, stand sideways in front of a mirror and adjust your profile so your hips are tucked under you, bringing your belly button toward your spine. Just focusing on good posture will strengthen your back and buttock muscles and cause you to stand and sit straighter. Concentrate on maintaining this good posture while you warm up and even when you are tired.

Your running technique will inevitably change as your body does—the key is to feel comfortable with and accept the changes. You will notice that lifting your feet off the ground becomes harder later in pregnancy and your stride becomes shorter, so your "run" may start to look like a shuffle. That's okay; just look out for tripping hazards.

If you feel out of breath or too hot while running, slow first to a brisk walk and then to a slow walk to bring your heart rate down. Keep track of your pace: you are getting a good workout if you are breathing hard but can still carry on a conversation.

Cooling Down

Always cool down for five minutes after your workout by walking slowly, then doing some stretching while your muscles are still warm. Stretching will help prevent muscle soreness and help you stay flexible for delivery. Pay particular attention to stretching the muscles in your legs: the hamstrings, quadriceps, and calves. If you find that your ankles become swollen after jogging, sit down and elevate your feet after you cool down, to get that extra blood to circulate back to your heart.

Equipment Considerations

If you have a good pair of running shoes from your pre-pregnancy jogs, they will serve you well throughout pregnancy and well after. However, you may find that shoes become a bit tighter as your feet swell later in pregnancy; try lacing them more loosely. You may even need shoes that are a half size bigger, especially if you exercise later in the day when your feet are more likely to be swollen. Lacing may be the other challenge during your third trimester. Cross-training shoes with Velcro straps, or shoes with no laces, will be easiest to get on and off. Lace locks, little plastic devices that secure your laces so you don't have to retie them, also work well. Just don't compromise your stability by heading out in nonrunning shoes!

Wearing a good bra is also important. Your most comfortable, supportive bra will work, or try wearing two sports bras for extra support. As your breasts grow, a bra with molded cups that aren't abrasive to your nipples will make you much more comfortable and will help you maintain a good posture. Similarly, if the bouncing is uncomfortable for your belly, a maternity belt can give you extra support. If abrasion of your upper thighs is bothering you, try cycling shorts (they'll stretch over your belly) or mesh nylon shorts that cover your thighs.

Preparing for Difficult Situations

If you're running a familiar route, take the usual safety precautions, such as using sunscreen and wearing a reflective vest in the evening. If you are away from your home turf, consider local hazards, such as heat and humidity or windchill. Exposure to vehicle exhaust or a change in altitude can also make you feel unusually worn out. Listen to your body and take a few days to get used to the new conditions before you start running again.

Planning Pointers for Pregnancy

1 Make your "run" a "run-walk." If you are an experienced runner, you will be able to continue running early in pregnancy, but take extra time to warm up and cool down. As your pregnancy progresses, make run-walking a more significant part of your routine, until you are walking briskly for half an hour at a time. If you've never been a runner, stick to walking during this pregnancy—so that you build your stamina without straining yourself.

2 Keep up your good habit. The more often you exercise, the easier the workout will be and the more energy you'll have. Establish a regular schedule for running or walking at least three times a week. Even if you don't feel up to running, you'll get a good workout if you walk and you'll appreciate the opportunity to unwind.

3 Pick comfortable gear. Use your running shoes for jogging and brisk walking because they give you the most support and stability. Choose a supportive bra that doesn't irritate you. Carry a small backpack with water, even for a short run.

4 Run with a buddy. You'll enjoy the run more and be safer in case of a problem if you're with someone. Plus, carrying on a conversation will help you moderate your pace.

5 Avoid the heat. Avoid running outside on hot or humid days. Always choose routes with shade and take frequent breaks, especially if you are heading uphill.

6 Warm up and cool down. You will simply be unable to carry on a run-walk routine if you don't warm up and cool down—you'll be too sore and achy. Use your warm-up to adjust your posture so that you avoid unnecessary strain on your back, hips, and shoulders.

7 Put safety first. Take a cell phone or at least some change for a pay phone in case you need help. Stay in well-traveled areas during your third trimester.

8 Enjoy yourself. Running, jogging, and run-walking will keep you in great shape and give you confidence in your changing body. Take advantage of your routine to enjoy the outdoors, get some time for yourself, take the dog out, and spend time with friends. As a result, you'll gain more energy for other tasks while conditioning your body for the marathon of labor and motherhood.

biking

If you are an experienced biker, cycling is a good way to stay in shape, especially during the first and second trimesters. Balancing shouldn't be a problem for you, since your center of gravity changes slowly, giving you time to adapt. On the other hand, if you feel wobbly on a bike or intimidated behind the handlebars, stick with an activity that doesn't involve balancing between two narrow wheels. If you thought balancing on a bike was hard a few months ago, try doing it while carrying a kicking and somersaulting fetus!

Biking buffs will recall the stories of the late national-team racer Miji Reoch, who biked throughout pregnancy (she even won criteriums in her first trimester) and, as legend has it, pedaled herself to the hospital while having labor contractions. This is not the approach I encourage you to take. Caution and awareness of your body's limits should guide your biking these nine months. Big-time racers learn to ignore signals of fatigue and injury when training. During pregnancy, however, attune yourself to those gentle reminders of your body's needs—your growing fetus depends on it.

If you've got a regular bike group you train with, stick with it as long as you are not sprinting or racing and can slow your pace if you have to. Remember to let your body, not your buddies or your ambitious fitness goals, set your limits. If you are a serious biker, you may have to change your fitness and weight expectations. You were probably above your racing weight when you conceived (you need that fat to get your estrogen levels up) and you need to continue to gain a healthy amount of weight throughout pregnancy. Don't worry—getting back in the saddle after delivery will help you shed those pounds quickly.

Feel free to continue riding occasionally on local bike routes or enjoying a brief bike commute to work—on safe paths—through your fifth or sixth month. If you have been an avid road biker who gets a rush from tackling steep hills or clocking fifty miles in an afternoon, you'll need to slow down and play it safer. Avoid big groups, pace lines, interval training, and racing. Think safety for two: be extra cautious about traffic and riding in control.

As your belly grows, sitting comfortably and being safe on a bicycle become more of a challenge. Plus, if you fall or are in an accident, your fetus is more vulnerable to injury. For this reason, I don't recommend road biking during your third trimester unless you are a very confident and experienced rider and stick to safe paths.

A good bike routine requires a safe, level bike path where you can relax instead of worrying about traffic, in-line skaters, or intersections. Always wear a helmet, choose your routes carefully, and seek out bike-only paths, such as rails-to-trails conversions (old train lines that have been converted to walking or biking trails). Remember, this is your time to unwind.

Biking is excellent aerobic exercise, since a half-hour bike ride will warm up your muscles and condition your heart and lungs. As soon as you break a sweat, you know you're getting a good workout and improving your chances of having an intervention-free delivery. Biking can also make your pregnancy easier by helping to prevent nausea, leg cramps, elevated blood sugars, and fatigue. Plus, the exercise will boost your energy, help you sleep better, and make you feel good about your changing body. Biking is not a weight-bearing exercise, however, so it does not have the same bone-strengthening benefits as running or hiking. Mix up your weekly workout activities to maximize the benefits for your pregnancy.

A half-hour total workout three times a week is very healthy for you and your baby. Warm up by coasting along slowly (or walking around) for five minutes to activate your muscles, then do some dynamic stretching so your back, calves, and arms are also ready to work and help maintain your posture (see chapter 6). Bike for twenty minutes (or up to an hour if you are taking it very easy), then cool down by coasting for another five before stretching out those still-warm muscles. You want to bike long enough to break a sweat, but avoid getting too hot or short of breath.

RISK ASSESSMENT BY TRIMESTER

1ST TRIMESTER: LOW

2ND TRIMESTER: MEDIUM

3RD TRIMESTER: MEDIUM

Staying Healthy Each Trimester

1ST TRIMESTER | RISK: LOW

As long as you are a confident biker, cycling occasionally or routinely during your first trimester is safe and good for your aerobic fitness. You'll also have a great time and maybe even reduce your nausea and improve your appetite. Sound good? Bike on!

biking

Because biking is easier (and more fun, for some) than running, you may be more enthusiastic about biking than about running during your first trimester even though your energy is low. Good for you: if you can keep up a regular biking routine, you'll be building your stamina and staying fit. And if you're biking simply as an excuse to get outside, biking on a flat path will allow you to exercise, talk with biking buddies, and enjoy the scenery while covering a good deal more distance than you would walking or running.

Instead of setting distance goals, think about the amount of time you want to be active, including time for warming up and cooling down. Thirty minutes is a good starting place, including five minutes of warming up, twenty minutes of biking, and five minutes of cooling down. Slowly work up to biking for half an hour on easy routes.

If you are an experienced cyclist, you'll be surprised at how much your training routine is affected by pregnancy. Start by cutting your training schedule in half. Then pare it down further as your growing pregnancy affects your stamina. Monitor yourself by paying attention to your breath—stop or slow down when you feel breathless.

Cutting down on your routine won't reduce your workout intensity, however. Most likely, you'll be drenched in sweat and thinking about turning around soon after the warm-up. That's okay: just slow down, avoid the big hills, and head home before you get too worn out. If you do hit a hill, you have permission to just get off the bike and walk, taking breaks to catch your breath.

The most important thing this trimester is to stay cool so that your fetus doesn't overheat. This means drinking plenty of water—I recommend carrying at least two bottles on your bike or a full water carrier on your back. Also, prehydrate: drink two glasses of water an hour before you start biking (and make sure to empty your bladder before heading out). Take off layers of clothing as you warm up and avoid going out at all if it's too hot, humid, or if your route would put you entirely in the sun on a warm day. Generally, take it easy and practice cruising.

If you feel comfortable biking regularly this trimester, you'll be in great shape to stay active throughout your pregnancy—even if you decide to switch to a stationary bike when the weather forces you indoors. Plus, you'll have more energy and a better attitude, which will help you get through this tiring trimester.

Something about biking during pregnancy made me feel really empowered—even more so than when I had pushed myself to work harder and go farther before pregnancy. Just getting on the saddle (and getting off my feet), feeling the familiar rhythm, and having that time alone felt good. Knowing that I could be active and foster the growth of my baby in utero was a powerful experience.

What surprised me the most was that I had to meet my body's demands, rather than just pushing through hunger, thirst, and fatigue as I had done before pregnancy. I think the transition is harder for women who have a high level of fitness. It's hard to let go of our notions of what it means to be fit and what constitutes an adequate workout.

I found ways to channel my extra energy toward my pregnancy instead of intense exercise. For example, the mental concentration I had reserved for pumping uphill at the lactate threshold, I instead focused on my growing baby. And, when it came to labor, I found myself thinking of contractions as hill repeats.

Several other biking moms had told me that I would be in terrific shape after delivery, although this was hard to believe since I felt like I hadn't left the couch in weeks. But it was true. Only two weeks after delivery, with my episiotomy scar still healing (apparently we bikers have bigger babies), I hit the road and felt great. I guess pregnancy and labor were sort of intensive training in themselves.

—Rosa, Corpus Christi, Texas

biking

You'll probably have a lot more energy to burn and still be pretty balanced and comfortable on a bike this trimester. Your belly is not quite big enough to keep you off a bike yet, although your fetus is now growing up into your abdomen and could get injured if you fall. More likely, the sudden impact of a fall can disrupt your placenta, causing a placental *abruption*, or tear, and endangering the fetus. Falling and accidents should be your biggest concerns, making road biking somewhat risky this trimester.

Well-conditioned cyclists will be loath to give up biking right when their energy kicks back in. For an experienced biker on a safe route, cycling can still be a good method of exercise. The key here is to make sure that your workout stays aerobic. During training or racing, when you push yourself beyond the comfort zone, your workout becomes anaerobic (meaning there simply isn't enough oxygen to feed your pumping muscles), and you end up with a buildup of lactic acid (which makes your muscles feel crampy) and total exhaustion. This period of low oxygen affects another muscle: your uterus. Anaerobic conditions limit the uterus's ability to deliver oxygen to the fetus, which can affect your fetus's organ development and growth.

The nice thing about biking is that it takes most of the load of your pregnancy off your legs and is easier on your joints than running. But that narrow little bike seat and your tender pelvis are supporting your weight. Sure, it's easier on your legs, but, believe me, your crotch (which is engorged with blood and more sensitive during pregnancy) will complain later if you don't have a comfortable seat and don't take frequent breaks to move around and get the blood flowing again.

This trimester, you may want to ramp up your gentle workout to include some hills. Your increased stamina this trimester may also allow you to bike longer distances and bike more often. Aim for a half-hour ride plus ten minutes of warming up and ten of cooling down at least three times a week. If cycling is your primary exercise, use the first half of the ride to break a sweat and get your heart rate up a bit, and the second half to gently work your muscles on a hill or in a higher gear; just don't push yourself too hard.

3RD TRIMESTER | RISK: MEDIUM

At this point, you can feel and even *see* the shape of your baby right below the surface of your belly. As your mothering instincts kick in, your baby will kick you to remind you to be cautious this trimester.

Unfortunately, there just isn't a helmet you can strap onto that belly. Imagine braking abruptly and hitting the handlebars with your belly, or skidding sideways and having the bike land on top of you, or, worse, being involved in an accident with a car. It's not just you who will be bruised and battered; it could mean bad news for your developing fetus. I advise choosing your bike route with caution (look for paths reserved for cyclists and pedestrians) or trying a stationary bike. And think about taking up another outdoor activity that you can enjoy for the rest of your pregnancy, like hiking.

If you climb on a bike this trimester, you'll find that your big belly simply gets in the way of pedaling as your knees bump your uterus. Even leaning forward slightly to hold the handlebars can put a lot of pressure on your lower abdomen, especially as your baby settles into the pelvis. I promise you'll enjoy biking a lot more when your baby is riding in a bike seat behind you.

If you just don't want to give up your biking routine, I recommend trying an indoor recumbent bike. These bikes allow you to recline so that you are not crowding your uterus and they also have comfortable, wide seats so you don't get a sore crotch. A half hour on a recumbent bike three times a week—especially if you program in a few inclines—is a terrific workout.

You may have a surprise in store for you when you get back on the bike after delivery, even after taking an extended break from biking. As one pro-cycling mother puts it, it's the phenomenon of the "über-mommies": after relatively lazy second and third trimesters and a few weeks of post-delivery recovery, this mom found that she developed six-pack abs and upped her racing class when she took up training again, As many fit women discover, pregnancy and the rigors of delivery had left her supercharged and more fit than ever.

biking

Warming Up

Warm up by biking a flat area or by simply walking around for five minutes. As soon as your legs feel a little warm, get off the bike for a couple of minutes to do some dynamic stretching to activate specific muscle groups (see chapter 6). Focus on your legs, calves, arms, and back. I know it's tempting to just keep on riding, but pausing to stretch will help prevent injuries and soreness down the road. Plus, warming up your arms and back will help you keep good posture on the bike.

Biking Technique for Pregnancy

If you're a confident biker, you probably discarded your training wheels decades ago and mastered no-hands riding in grade school. Your confidence will serve you well, but let caution guide your riding during pregnancy. Unless you're a racer, you probably rarely think about your technique or biking posture. Maybe you aren't even clear on how to adjust the height of your seat or handlebars. This is the time to learn.

The first thing to watch is your posture: good posture will save you from some major back soreness. The most important rule is to keep your back as straight as possible. As with sitting or standing, arching your back or hunching over strains your back muscles. Even though you are leaning forward a little, keep your shoulders and hips aligned—imagine a string running from your neck to your tailbone. As you get tired, and especially when your pregnancy gets a little bigger, you will tend to arch your back so that your lower back caves inward toward your belly. As you're riding, make a mental note to check on your back and adjust your position. And when you get off the bike to take breaks, stretch your back (try clasping your fingers together, palms out, and straightening them in front of you, to lengthen those back muscles) so it doesn't surprise you later with some serious aching.

The second thing to keep in mind is your relationship to the handlebars. It's not just a matter of holding on to them—the angle at which you grasp the handlebars will completely affect your position on the bike. If you ride occasionally or have a cruise bike or a hybrid mountain-road bike, you probably have your handlebars adjusted so that you sit pretty upright on the bike. This is good. On the other hand, if you have a racing road bike or have your handlebars adjusted low, then you are leaning far forward onto the handlebars. This is really aerodynamic, but it's no fun for your uterus, which can get really cramped. Plus, it can add to the strain on your back. Very early in your pregnancy, you'll still be comfortable in your usual bike position, but as your uterus grows and your crotch becomes more sensitive (around your third month of pregnancy), you'll need to adjust your seat and handlebars so that you can sit up nearly straight while still extending your legs when pedaling. You can probably make the adjustments yourself, or just take your bike in to a bike shop and have them fix it for you.

Pace yourself along the way so that you don't get too hot or out of breath. Remember, it's okay to hop off and walk or stop if you need to. If you're talking and having fun, you're going just the right speed. A healthy pace allows you to breathe deeply but still carry on a conversation—and enjoy the view.

Cooling Down

Don't abruptly stop exercising at the top of a grueling hill—take five minutes to cool down first, either by walking or biking on level ground. Take advantage of your warm muscles to stretch and maintain your flexibility, which is important for an easier delivery. Concentrate on stretching the muscles you just used: the hamstrings, quadriceps, and calves.

Equipment Considerations

There are few absolutes when it comes to exercising safely and here is one of them: if you don't have a helmet, stay off your bike. Some accidents are simply unavoidable, and it's so easy to slap on a helmet and protect yourself from a serious head injury. Your baby is going to need you with your head squarely on your shoulders—don't take chances with it.

If you don't already have a helmet, go pick one up and choose one that is comfortable and doesn't move a lot when you shake your head. Look for snazzy reflectors and lights too. As you well know, a bike is easy for drivers to miss, even in broad daylight, even when you have right of way, and even when you're in the designated bike lane. You want to do everything you can to make yourself as visible as possible, even if it means wearing one of those not-so-chic mesh reflective vests to protect you and your baby.

biking

For stability, consider riding a hybrid or mountain bike, even on paved paths, or putting wider tires on your road bike. The more upright frame of a mountain or hybrid bike will be easier to ride later in pregnancy; you may even decide to temporarily replace your regular handlebar stem with an upright tourist stem for maximum comfort. For safety, ride without toe clips and straps and put away those clipless pedals during pregnancy. You want to be able to quickly put your feet down for balance in order to prevent falls.

The increase in the hormone relaxin means that your joints are looser and more susceptible to carpal tunnel syndrome during pregnancy. Wearing padded gloves and frequently shifting your hand position can help relieve wrist strain.

One great thing about your bike is that it can carry your water for you. Just make sure you have a water bottle holder (or two) and full bottles of water; you won't even have to stop cruising along to grab a drink. Also, think about taking a bike lock with you, in case you decide you're happier walking—then you can lock up your bike, walk to your destination, and get it on the way back.

If you've never had a good relationship with your bike seat, now may be the time to invest in a more comfortable padded saddle. The wide, molded seats cradle your buttocks and are the most comfortable when riding longer distances, but you can also try the seats that elevate you onto your sitting bones and have a little indent in the middle and gel padding. Yes, these seats were originally designed for protecting testicles, but they can relieve soreness in women too. Many women find these seats particularly comfortable after delivery when the vaginal area and episiotomy sutures are still healing.

You'll be glad to know that those stretchy spandex bike shorts you may already own will stretch right around your belly and help prevent abrasion of your inner thighs with pedaling. Plus, if you get shorts with some padding built into the crotch, you'll be able to tolerate that seat longer.

Preparing for Difficult Situations

Your toughest situation on the bike is going to be dealing with traffic. My advice, in short, is to stay away from it. I recommend sticking to designated bike paths—especially if they are totally separate from car traffic, like in a park—and quiet roads with bike lanes. Bike-friendly cities produce maps highlighting bike routes, and the local outdoors outfitter can also give you some pointers. Many parks have paved service roads that are level and don't see any cars or many pedestrians.

Plan a round-trip route that is bicycle-friendly so that you don't end up on some busy streets unintentionally. Breathing a lot of exhaust and dust, riding alongside trucks or fast-moving traffic, or being shoved onto a narrow or unpaved shoulder can ruin your ride and be downright dangerous. If you plan ahead and pay attention to the rules of the road—and that means using hand signals before turning and calling out before passing pedestrians—you'll be in pretty good shape for avoiding mishaps.

Even though you're wearing a helmet, don't forget to protect your face and other exposed parts with sunscreen. And don't take off that helmet, even if you're sweating buckets—just get out of the sun and off the bike for a break. In the event that you're still out when the temperature drops in the evening, tie an extra sweatshirt or long-sleeved t-shirt around your waist.

Planning Pointers for Pregnancy

1 Bike with confidence. If you love riding, go for it! Enjoy the fresh air, exercise, and exhilaration, but let caution guide you. If you don't feel stable on a bike or just aren't an experienced biker, stick to an activity that you can enjoy with confidence.

2 Plan a bicycle-friendly route. Pick up a local map of bike routes and explore the area to figure out where the bike paths are before taking out your bike. Throw a bike rack on your car and drive to a bike path. For a relaxing ride, stick to parks and bike-only routes.

3 Know your limits. It's exciting to embark on a long ride, conquer a big hill, and scream down an endless slope—but it's important to listen to your body during pregnancy. Plan a slower pace, shorter distance, more breaks, and flexible return time. Remember, your goal is to have fun—not train for the Tour de France.

4 Helmet. Helmet. Helmet. Don't ride your bike without it.

5 Ride with a buddy. Riding while having a conversation will help you pace yourself and will make your ride fly by. Plus, you'll have help—just in case.

6   Fill your tank. You lose tons of water when biking because of the exercise, the heat, and the wind drying your skin. So prehydrate and keep your bike loaded with plenty of water. You can even try freezing one of your water bottles so that when it melts en route you'll have cool water on your way back.

7   Stay cool. Choose routes with shade and take frequent breaks, especially if you are heading uphill.

8   Warm up and sit straight. It's easy to forget to warm up once you climb on your bike, so reserve a little extra time to walk around first or bike on a flat path for five minutes to a turnout where you can pause for some stretching. During your warm-up, focus on your posture. Make sure that when you sit on your bike your back is flat and you are sitting almost upright.

9   Enjoy your ride. Biking is a great way to enjoy the outdoors and stay in shape. Plus, it's one activity that you'll be able to share with your baby early on—and she'll love it as much as you do!

in-line skating

In-line skating or ice skating are embraced by outdoor enthusiasts who love speed and want a fun way to get around without a lot of hassle. Anywhere there is a paved path, you'll find in-line skaters. You probably know of a neighborhood park that is whizzing every weekend with energetic converts to the sport. It is fantastic exercise, great transportation, and not too hard to learn—especially if you've got a knack for roller skating, ice skating, or even skiing.

What about in-line (or ice) skating during pregnancy? If you are a confident and cautious skater, keep it up during your first trimester—that is, if you really know how to turn, stop, and avoid obstacles. Skating is as good an aerobic exercise as jogging—but it has a much higher risk of falls. And you'll be falling on solid asphalt (or ice). If you're just starting out, are pretty unsteady on skates and still take some scrapes, or just haven't mastered the trick of stopping, hang up the blades until after the baby's born. It just won't be any fun enduring a broken wrist or a concussion along with the other symptoms of pregnancy—and you certainly don't want to endanger your baby by having a serious injury (although during the first trimester the fetus is protected because the uterus is safely tucked behind the pubic bone). Pregnancy is not a good time to learn to skate, experiment with new tricks, or join an ice hockey team. Racing or competitive games make it more likely you'll get injured badly. And stay away from hills.

In-line and ice skating are endurance sports, which means that they build the strength of your heart and lungs. Skating regularly during your first trimester will keep you in good shape and build your stamina for labor and delivery and for all your day-to-day activities during pregnancy. If you're in good shape, you'll be less winded and have more energy. Skating also strengthens your lower back and legs, the muscles you rely on the most to carry your growing pregnancy.

The good news is that skating during your first trimester will make your second trimester easier. In-line or ice skating regularly will help control varicose veins, elevated blood sugars, and leg cramps. It will help you sleep better and feel more confident about your changing body. Plus, if you skate your first trimester (and have a good time doing it), you'll be much more likely to stay active for the rest of your pregnancy. When you begin your second trimester, simply switch to jogging, biking, or walking. You'll see the same parks at a whole different pace—and you'll still get a good workout and enjoy your time outdoors.

RISK ASSESSMENT BY TRIMESTER

    1ST TRIMESTER: MEDIUM

    2ND TRIMESTER: HIGH

    3RD TRIMESTER: HIGH

Staying Healthy Each Trimester

1ST TRIMESTER | RISK: MEDIUM

It can be difficult to keep up a regular exercise routine during the first trimester, when your body may feel out of sorts. That's why it is so important to choose activities that you really want to do—so that you're motivated to stay active. If your trusty blades are calling to you to get out and do something, go for it.

Skating is great exercise and a lot of fun, as long as you know what you are doing. If you are confident in your skating skills—and you have all the right safety gear—then you are set to hit some flat, smooth, well-lighted paths or a skating rink. But even if you were a championship roller skater in the sixth grade and have mastered the roller-slalom course, skating is still pretty risky. Wearing skates gives you extra height, so it's a long way to topple. And there are a lot of unpredictable factors: like potholes, traffic, and unruly walkers. Keep your eyes open and use caution while skating.

Decide how long you want to be out rather than how far you want to skate. Don't forget to set aside time to warm up and cool down. Getting too hot or worn out right now is not good for your fetus's development. That means carrying a water bottle and drinking about a liter per hour of exercise. Wear layers so that you can unpeel them as you warm up and rest in the shade if you feel too hot.

Warm up by coasting five minutes, then do some dynamic stretching—yes, you can do this on wheels or on ice skates, if you're careful—to warm up your arms, back, and legs (see chapter 6). Strong arms and back will help you maintain a good posture and balance so that you don't injure yourself or fall. Skate for about twenty minutes (gradually increasing to forty minutes as you get in better shape or if you are taking it very easy), so that you break a sweat and get your heart pumping. Cool down by coasting for another five. Then take off your skates and stretch while your muscles are still warm. A total workout of skating for at least half an hour three days a week will keep you in great shape.

in-line skating

2ND TRIMESTER | RISK: HIGH

As your fetus grows up into your belly, it becomes more vulnerable to injury. At the same time, you become considerably less stable on your feet—let alone on a row of wheels or a thin ice-skate blade. And even your helmet and top-of-the-line safety gear won't protect your uterus if you take a tumble.

At this stage any fall—even if it's not directly onto your belly—can affect your fetus. Say, for example, you lose control skating around a corner and fall onto your bottom. In that instant, your fetus is thrown against the top of the uterus and the delicate placenta is wrenched forward, causing serious damage to the the fetus's blood supply. So even if you still feel stable on in-line skates or ice skates during your third month of pregnancy, I don't recommend skating after your first trimester—a fall would be too risky for your pregnancy.

Trade in the wheels for a solid pair of shoes. Hiking, brisk walking, or snow shoeing will give you as good a workout as skating did, without the risk of falling—or being crashed into. Plus, hiking is an outdoor activity you can keep up through the end of your pregnancy.

3RD TRIMESTER | RISK: HIGH

By your third trimester, you won't even consider lacing up your skates—you won't even be able to see your feet. Imagine trying to keep your balance and maintain good posture on skates! If it's not entirely impossible, it is certainly not a good idea. That doesn't mean you should stick to the rocking chair. Try walking instead. You'll get an excellent workout, won't fall, and you'll maintain your stamina for delivery.

Warming Up

After lacing up, warm up by cruising a flat area. This will get your blood pumping and prepare your muscles for a little stretching. Then find a quiet spot where you can stretch (see below) for a couple of minutes—a grassy patch or an empty part of the rink is useful.

Wearing your skates, try these simple stretches after warming up. Grab an ankle and pull it back toward your buttock to stretch your upper leg (quadriceps) muscles. Release. Lift that foot forward and do some ankle circles (this will be harder if your boots are laced tightly). Then straighten the leg and lift it behind

"When I first learned to skate in high school, it meant transportation and freedom. It wasn't so easy to learn—I used the collision-stopping technique for several years—but I've been skating regularly for more than ten years now and gliding, turning, and slowing down have become second nature. When I became pregnant, skating was a part of my life, and I couldn't imagine giving it up for nine months or more. So I decided to continue skating as long as I felt comfortable with it and could do it safely.

What a wonderful feeling it is to glide along when you are pregnant! The back pain and discomfort disappeared. I felt like I could be myself. I was happy to be able to enjoy my usual outdoor activities even though I was pregnant.

During my first trimester, ice skating season started. Here in Sweden, long-distance ice skating is very popular. People use ice skates with longer, thinner blades and skate out on large lakes and on the ocean when it freezes over. My husband is an avid skater too so we try to get out on the ice as many times as we can.

I noticed that many of my friends who have been pregnant felt a bit victimized by the whole experience and cut way back on their own interests simply because they felt big and sort of handicapped. Skating helped me overcome those feelings of being trapped inside my own body. It's truly wonderful.

—Emily, Stockholm, Sweden"

you to activate the buttocks (gluteus) muscles and the backs of your legs (hamstrings). Repeat on the other side. While standing straight, rotate your hips around in five gentle circles to your right, then to your left. Hip circles will warm up your hips and lower back. Don't forget to warm up your back, shoulders, and arms with dynamic stretches, which activate your muscles so that you can maintain good posture and balance when skating (see chapter 6).

In-Line Skating Technique for Pregnancy

Posture is key to stable, safe skating. You'll notice that a master skater stays low to the ground, with her back flat and her knees bent. It's simple: the lower your center of gravity, the less likely you are to fall.

Good technique requires keeping your leg and back muscles strong so that you are confident in your movements. Between skating excursions, maintain that leg strength by doing supported squats and lunges—*without* your skates on. Build your belly, back, and buttocks muscles by doing hip lifts to activate the abdominal muscles. Then focus on your posture when you skate. Even though you are leaning forward when you are moving, keep your shoulders straight—not hunched—and your back flat—not arched. Keep your weight balanced over the balls of your feet and your feet four to six inches apart. If you lock your knees while moving, you are almost guaranteed to fall. I promise that practicing good skating posture will give you excellent standing and sitting posture as well and will really support your back as your pregnancy grows.

Cooling Down

It's easy to forget to cool down when you've finally arrived back at the car or your front porch—you'll probably just want to pull off those skates and take a shower. Well, if you haven't already cooled down by cruising on flat ground for five minutes to get your heart rate down, you need to do it now. Or take off the skates and walk around in your socks for five minutes as your breathing returns to normal. Then try some pregnancy-safe stretches.

Equipment Considerations

Skating equipment is all about safety. And it works really well for you during your first trimester. Unfortunately, there is just no gear that can protect your growing belly after that. As soon as you put on your skates, you'll notice the increased distance to the ground. As you probably learned the first time you skated, it's no fun to fall that far. During pregnancy, you are more likely to bruise and sprain. So you need all the safety equipment you can get. Well-fitting skates that lace up and support your ankles should be at the top of your list. Broken wrists are the most common skating injury. Wrist guards support your delicate wrists. Knee and elbow pads can save your skin. A long-sleeved shirt and a pair of jeans also help protect your skin. Don't even consider skating without a snug-fitting helmet. Wear it low on your head, about an inch above your eyebrows. Avoid skating at dusk, when you are hard to see—or wear a headlamp and reflective jacket to get drivers' and bikers' attention.

Preparing for Difficult Situations

Your most difficult situation is going to be negotiating roads. Traffic laws treat in-line skating as a recreational activity that falls somewhere between biking and walking. You are often allowed on sidewalks, but you have to yield to pedestrians. The best places to skate are paths in parks where there are few walkers and bikers. Empty parking lots, basketball courts, and tennis courts also provide nice, smooth surfaces for a skating workout. On ice skates, stick to less-trafficked parts of the rink and skate with the flow.

Planning Pointers for Pregnancy

1 Skate with confidence. If you are an experienced skater and love an afternoon of whizzing by the scenery, keep it up during your first trimester. After your third month, however, a fall could endanger your pregnancy, so hang up the skates until after delivery.

2 Plan a skater-friendly route. Uncrowded and paved walking trails are the best locations. A crowded sidewalk or a bike lane alongside speeding cars just isn't safe—or relaxing.

3 Take it easy. Skating allows you to really enjoy the scenery and cover some distance while getting a good workout. Forget the roller or ice hockey, showy tricks, and downhill roller slalom. This is your time to meditate.

4 Helmet. Helmet. Helmet. Never skate without it.

5 Talk and skate. Chatting with a friend while skating will make the time fly by—and it can help you monitor your exertion. If you're breathing deeply but still talking comfortably, you're going the right speed.

6 Drink up—often. As you glide by those huffing and puffing joggers, you may not realize that you're getting just as good a workout—and sweating just as much—as they are. You need to replace your fluids. Carry water on you (try a hip carrier) or plan your route to include stops at water fountains.

7 Skate cool. No, that doesn't mean wearing hot pants and a bandanna. It means keeping your temperature down. Choose paths with shade and take breaks, especially if you are heading uphill.

8 Think posture. Regular skating will do wonders for your posture—on skates and off. And the strong back muscles you build while skating are especially good for preventing backaches later on in pregnancy.

9 It's supposed to be fun. If you didn't love skating so much, you'd be swimming laps in a prenatal class, right? So find your stride and enjoy yourself.

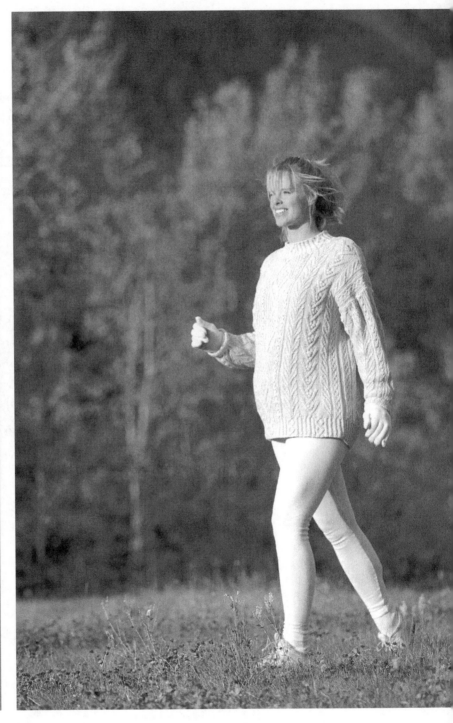

chapter 9

Staying Active in the Woods

We long to get outdoors to experience fresh air, peace and quiet, and adventure. For many of us, this means heading to the woods. Whether at a nearby trail or a cherished national park, visiting the wilderness brings balance into our active lives.

Some of your favorite places may be in the woods: a flower-strewn meadow discovered on a backpacking trip, a biking trail with countless stream crossings, or a camping spot with a view of the ocean. But the wilderness may be no farther away than a stroll off the pavement. There, we can watch birds, cast for fish, track wildlife, identify wildflowers, and nourish our souls.

When you're pregnant, it may be even more important for you to get away from it all. But heading into the wilderness during pregnancy raises a few concerns. The roughness of the terrain, the altitude, and the remoteness of your location become important considerations. If you hike, camp, mountain bike, mountaineer, or horseback ride, you'll need to consider the possible risks carefully before heading out into the wilderness. And you'll want to be prepared with the right gear. Your excursion should be as comfortable for you as it is safe for your fetus. Soon enough, you'll share your love of the woods with that curious youngster.

hiking

Hiking is a great way to get outdoors, whether in a local park or in the remote backcountry. Bring a topographic map and really explore, or bring your toddler and take it easy: the challenge is up to you. Just pick a place you want to see and reserve at least half an hour to really enjoy it. Getting out in nature may have special significance to you during pregnancy since your own body is buzzing with the force of its reproductive energy. There isn't anything routine about hiking, even if you do the same trail over and over again—it will always show you something new. Whether you're already an outdoor buff or you're just thinking about getting more active during pregnancy, you'll probably enjoy hiking.

And it's a really good workout. Hiking is both safe and distracting—two essential qualities in an exercise routine during pregnancy. Hiking up and down hills gives your entire body a good workout and is relatively easy on your joints and muscles. Hiking is not only an aerobic exercise, which works out your heart and lungs, it is also a weight-bearing exercise. This means that simply carrying your body weight during hiking works your muscles, joints, and bones. The more weight you carry, whether it is a backpack or the pregnancy itself, the greater your workout.

Even better, if you hike regularly during pregnancy, you reap the many benefits of being fit, including having fewer aches and pains, a better body image, and an enhanced feeling of well-being. And unlike biking and swimming, which are not weight-bearing exercises, hiking also helps you maintain a healthy weight (and gain less fat) during later pregnancy, have a shorter labor, and experience fewer complications and interventions at birth.

Hiking is a relatively low-risk activity during pregnancy: you can feel confident that hiking is good for you and your baby. Let's be absolutely clear on one thing: hiking will not cause bleeding or other complications during pregnancy. As long as you listen to your body, stay hydrated, and take frequent breaks, you really can't go wrong. Just keep in mind that if you are feeling too hot, cold, or worn out, it's time to stop. Plan a hike that is moderately challenging, but don't overexert yourself.

If you were fairly inactive before pregnancy, hiking is an excellent way to start exercising—especially if you live near a scenic trail or can hike with someone (or your dog). The scenery will keep you motivated, so make your goal something you'll appreciate, like reaching a scenic spot or a lake.

RISK ASSESSMENT BY TRIMESTER

1ST TRIMESTER: LOW
2ND TRIMESTER: LOW
3RD TRIMESTER: MEDIUM

Staying Healthy Each Trimester

1ST TRIMESTER | RISK: LOW

If you hiked before pregnancy, you're probably in pretty good shape and it will be easier for you to stay active during your first trimester. Don't be surprised if you feel tired when you're just getting started. As with other weight-bearing exercise, you will notice that you have less stamina when hiking early in pregnancy. Don't get discouraged: this will get better. Nausea and morning sickness may also interfere with your plans: eat small snacks and drink lots of water so they don't hit you while on the trail. You may also find that the fresh air makes you feel better.

This trimester, the main thing you should watch out for is overexerting yourself. The fact that you don't look pregnant yet doesn't mean that you can handle all the steep trails and long distances you tackled a few months ago. Take it easy. Remember that overheating is not healthy for your fetus, so be sure to dress in removable layers and hike during cooler times of the day. If you start to heat up en route, take a break, head onto a flatter trail, and pace yourself.

When planning a hike this trimester, look for scenic routes rather than grueling summits. Often, creek-side trails are refreshing and less strenuous because they stick to a gently sloping valley. You are more sensitive to sunburn and dehydration, so pick a trail with shade. During the first six months or so of pregnancy, especially if you're an experienced hiker, you'll be able to tackle most terrain safely, including narrow, rocky trails and switchbacks. Keep an eye on altitude and avoid summits over eight thousand feet. If you're coming from near sea level, take time to acclimatize, even if you're only headed to three or four thousand feet elevation.

A hike that gets your heart pumping is good for you and your tiny developing fetus—and you won't endanger your pregnancy by hitting the trails as often as you can. Aim to hike for twenty minutes twice a week and take a longer

hiking

hike—at least an hour—once a week. If you are lucky enough to live near a hiking trail, you may be able to work in a morning or evening hike into your schedule during the week. On the weekend, grab your partner, your dog, your children, or a friend and explore new territory. Weekday hikes of a mile or two will keep you in shape for going on weekend excursions of three to five miles without any difficulty.

Hiking regularly—say at least three times a week—rather than sporadically, will help you avoid injury and enjoy the greatest health benefits. But you can mix and match your exercise activites: hiking can become your "default" activity if you want to get outdoors but don't feel up for gathering lots of equipment and don't have time to be out for more than an hour or two. Just keep your hiking shoes and sunscreen by the door and a map of nearby trails handy so that you get out as much as you can.

2ND TRIMESTER | RISK: LOW

You may really feel like getting out there this trimester. Well, go for it! With your nausea out of the way and a burst of energy at your disposal, you may be eager to enjoy a change of scenery. Hiking is an excellent option during the second trimester because it is easier on your joints than running and it is a quick and easy way to get outdoors. Plus, hiking, unlike most other exercise, really allows for good conversation, so it may also give you an opportunity to catch up with your loved ones.

If you didn't exercise much during your first trimester, hiking will allow you to get in shape gradually while enjoying the outdoors. Hiking is easy to take up during pregnancy because you can control your workout. It is easy on your joints, doesn't jolt your belly, allows for frequent and spontaneous breaks, and lets you focus on the scenery rather than on your workout. If you have been starting to think that keeping up your fitness level during pregnancy seems like a chore, hiking regularly will change your mind—and refresh your senses.

This trimester, pick trails that have gentle grades sufficient to get your heart pumping but are not so steep that you will injure yourself when descending. Keep in mind that your joints are more relaxed now, and slopes that were hard on your knees and ankles before pregnancy will be even tougher. Watch out for slippery stream crossings and muddy trails. As your belly grows and you have less visibility around your feet (you can't see them), avoid uneven paths and

Up until a month before my pregnancy, I was traveling through Asia and hiking in some of the most spectacular places on earth, like Nepal and Thailand. I felt so adventurous and carefree. When I got pregnant, I kept it up, just closer to home. My husband and I would make time on weekends to go somewhere really beautiful and get outdoors. Of course, I would get flushed, winded, and sweat more than usual and we would go about two miles in the time it used to take us to go six, but I felt really good about my health and my pregnancy—and I was in fantastic shape. And the best part: my husband let me pick the hikes!

About three months into my pregnancy, I started spotting and my midwife told me to stop exercising. She assured me that nothing I had done—not even the strenuous hikes—had caused the bleeding, but she wanted me to take it easy anyway. Following her advice, I stopped biking and running and I even walked much less. After a few weeks of feeling cooped up, I did join a prenatal yoga class—which I loved—but it didn't give me the rigorous workouts I had been used to.

Toward the end of my pregnancy, when it would be safe to go into labor, my midwife told me I could start hiking again. I just loved being back in the woods and looked forward to sharing it with my baby. We discovered a few parks close to home and I would lug my big body along on the flat trails where I didn't have to see where I was stepping—I couldn't see my feet anyway! But it was so worth it to be out there and have some peaceful time with my husband.

As my due date came and went, I hiked more and more, trying to encourage labor to start. I don't think the hiking helped bring on the labor but it sure helped me stay relaxed!

—Stacey, Olympia, Washington

rocky trails that require careful foot placement. Although your body may not be considerable wider, your gait and arm swing are more generous, so you may need to slow down on narrow passages or along cliffs to establish your balance.

Hiking a one- to two-mile loop twice a week will stretch your muscles and give you an aerobic boost. Round out the week with a three- to five-mile trail; aim to hike for at least ninety minutes. Since you'll have more energy this trimester, once or twice a month go on day hikes that get you outdoors for three or four hours at a time; depending on the heat, the altitude, your fitness level, and the elevation changes, these long hikes should be four to eight miles.

With a regular hiking regimen, you'll be in terrific shape, have a positive outlook, and spend time bonding with your hiking partner and your fetus. Exercising during your second trimester means you'll feel better during your third trimester as well.

3RD TRIMESTER | RISK: MEDIUM

You may have a little reality check your third trimester. Hikes that were easy earlier on in pregnancy may seem more difficult now. First, you're huffing and puffing from just the warm-up. Second, you're lugging this huge belly around. And third, you can't even see your feet to know where you're stepping!

However, you can pick easier hikes and still both get a good workout and get outdoors for a mental break. Simply carrying your pregnancy weight adds to the intensity of your aerobic and weight-bearing exercise. Even brief hikes build stamina, which many women find peaks around the sixth month.

You don't have to climb a mountain to get a good view. This trimester, pick trails that offer rewarding sights en route, like wildflowers, a meandering brook, or towering redwoods. This way, you can turn around early without feeling like you missed the finale.

As your belly grows, your ability to find safe footing diminishes, and rocky, muddy, or narrow paths become increasingly hazardous. Many national parks have trails that are designated "multi-use," meaning they are paved and wider than other trails. Also, look for service roads through parks and national forest land. These dirt or paved roads traverse the area with fewer obstacles and gentler grades. Rails-to-trails conversions are old train lines that have been turned into walking or biking trails. These are also excellent options this trimester, since rail beds make flat trails that are often far from traffic and accessible from urban areas.

You may develop back pain and pelvic discomfort after even a short hike late in pregnancy. Warming up and cooling down, even with a brief hike, is crucial: you're naturally carrying much more weight than usual, so the strain on your muscles and joints is more significant. Unlike a paved path, the graded terrain and unpredictable surface of a hiking trail demands good balance, quick reflexes, and flexibility; supportive shoes, a walking stick, and a thorough warm-up are your best preparation for these conditions.

After your hike and cooldown, take off your shoes, get off your feet, and elevate your legs to avoid ankle swelling. Regular hiking will help reduce chronic swelling and varicose veins by improving your legs' blood flow.

You may notice some Braxton Hicks contractions—or tightening across your belly—when you're hiking. This is common. It doesn't mean that you're going into labor: the contractions should go away when you rest for a few minutes. Even if you feel these irregular contractions every time you hike, they are not harmful to your baby. Don't let this "false labor" scare you into staying on your couch.

This trimester, aim to hike twice a week. One of those hikes can be a brief one-mile jaunt, plus ten minutes of warm-up and cooldown time. At this point in pregnancy, you may consider the hike itself the warm-up for a delicious, relaxed stretching session. Once a week, get outdoors for a longer hike. Aim for three miles; depending on the trail and your level of fitness, this may take a couple of hours. Remember to stick to well-trafficked areas or areas that have cell phone coverage and are easily reachable.

Warming Up

Begin your hike by walking on flat ground for five minutes. Then do some dynamic stretches to activate your legs, back, and hips (see chapter 6). Remember that warming up before getting out on the trail will help you prevent injuries and soreness. Plus, it'll keep you from becoming breathless when you hit that first hill.

Hiking Technique for Pregnancy

Posture is very important when hiking. You may not even notice your poor posture, but you'll certainly feel your aching back later. When hiking, keep your back straight and your shoulders relaxed. Keep your head up and look ahead of you: looking down can give you a sore back. Swing your arms from the shoulders and keep your elbows bent, with your hands at the level of your waist. When walking quickly or going uphill, lean slightly into the trail to shift your weight forward, but avoid bending at your waist, which can strain your back.

Your shifting center of gravity also affects your hiking posture and maneuverability. After the fifth or sixth month, you'll probably tend to arch your back and stick out your big belly. This can make it difficult to quickly change direction or come to a quick stop when walking—and it'll give you muscle pain. Before heading out, take a look at your profile in a mirror and practice tucking your pelvis under you so that your shoulders and hips are in line: this is how you should hold your back when you're hiking.

Keep track of the intensity of your hike as well. You are hiking at the right pace if you are breathing hard but are still able to carry on a conversation. If you are short of breath, slow it down. If you are doing a tough hike—like climbing a steep trail—take your pulse and make sure that you are keeping your heart rate below 140 beats per minute. On the other hand, if you are not getting enough of a workout (your heart rate is below 100 beats per minute), head uphill or take a longer hike.

Cooling Down

Slow your pace gradually to allow your heart rate to return to normal—walk a few laps around the parking lot before getting back in the car. Cooling down for at least ten minutes prevents a sudden drop in blood flow to the uterus when you stop exercising. Then take a few minutes to stretch while your muscles are warm, to boost flexibility and prevent soreness. If you find that your ankles become swollen after hiking, sit down and elevate your feet above the level of your heart after you cool down, to get that extra blood to circulate back to your heart. Postpone your shower for fifteen minutes so that your body has time to return blood flow to the uterus—the hot water will draw a lot of blood back to your skin and away from your internal organs (like during exercise).

Equipment Considerations

The great thing about hiking is that a solid pair of walking shoes and a bottle of water are all you really need to get started. Having a good pair of shoes can help keep you from slipping or losing your footing; those popular slip-ons just aren't going to do the trick. And supportive shoes will help prevent poor posture and muscle aches—both now and when you're carrying your baby in your arms. Keeping your water and snacks accessible is also key so that you stay well hydrated and maintain your blood sugar level while hiking.

The gear you are used to hiking with—a bulky backpack or fanny pack stuffed with snacks—may be uncomfortable during pregnancy. Instead, a smaller daypack—or hydration pack with room for snacks and a windbreaker—is ideal. A pack with hip straps also helps take the strain off your shoulders and back. If you want to enjoy your hike, just be sure you're comfortable with the gear you've got.

Preparing for Difficult Situations

Depending on where you are hiking, you may be faced with conditions that make the excursion more challenging—and possibly pose some risks to you and the fetus. Think about the length, intensity, terrain, remoteness, and rescue accessibility of your hike. Even if the trail is in a local park, you need to know the answers to the following questions: Are there shortcuts you could take if you needed to? Is the return trek uphill? Is the trail popular and well maintained? Are there restrooms and water fountains? Is there a park ranger who patrols the area? Are there muddy, rocky, or underwater parts of the trail? Is there shade?

If you're planning to try a wilderness trail—especially if it's remote—ask yourself: Will altitude be a concern? Am I prepared for weather changes while on the trail? Should I be concerned about insects and, worse, insect-borne diseases, like Lyme disease? Do I have enough water for the trip?

If you're well prepared, you can challenge yourself with confidence.

Planning Pointers for Pregnancy

1 Plan a shorter hike. Remember that your stamina is decreased during pregnancy, so plan a less rigorous hike. I recommend starting with a walk of a mile or two, especially if you haven't been very active. If you're a veteran hiker, six to eight miles should be your maximum. Choose a hike that will allow you to loop back early if you need to.

2 Make it a habit. The more often you hike, the better you'll feel on the trail and the rest of the day. If you feel up to it, work up to a regular schedule of hiking.

3 Adjust your equipment. Get footwear that offers good arch and ankle support, carry more water and snacks, and distribute weight among your hiking partners so you can carry less. (The less you carry, the easier it will be to stop for bathroom breaks.)

4 Stay on well-groomed trails. Follow easy-to-navigate trails where possible. Narrow trails with lots of rocks, loose gravel, and fallen trees can be hard to negotiate as your pregnancy progresses. You'll still get a good workout on a paved path—and you won't be so worried about losing your footing.

5 Hike with a buddy. It is safest, especially after your first trimester, to go with a friend in case of an emergency and to get help carrying your gear. If you're hiking alone, let someone know exactly where you are heading and when you plan to return, even if it's just for a few hours. Just leave a message on a friend's answering machine or a note for your partner at home.

6 Avoid the heat. Don't hike on hot or humid days, when you may overheat. Always choose shaded trails and take frequent breaks, especially if you are heading uphill and are sweating buckets.

7 Know how to get help. Choose trails that allow you to call for and get help if you need it, such as those with cell phone coverage, lots of other hikers, or a ranger patrol.

8 Remember to stop and smell the flowers. Hiking isn't just about the exercise; you're out there to clear your mind, explore a new place, and get some fresh air. When you pause to catch that view, take a deep breath and imagine sharing this with your baby.

camping

It can be hard to explain to a confirmed city-dweller why you would leave the comforts of your couch, bed, and hot shower to hang around a smoky fire, sleep on the ground, and wake to frost. But if you love the outdoors, the attraction is clear: the satisfaction of building a fire and cooking outdoors, the coziness of a sleeping bag, and the awesome night sky. You'll never forget the morning you caught a moose at your picnic table or the midnight you woke to a chorus of howling wolves. Camping brings us closer to nature, to our instincts, and, yes, even to each other. A camping excursion while pregnant can be wonderful—especially if the sun is shining, the river looks inviting, and the mosquitoes have left town.

We each have our own definition of camping. For some, it's a full-fledged backpacking trip with dried food, pack-out trash bags, and one change of underwear. For others, it means an RV with a refrigerator, four solid walls, and even a satellite TV. Between these two extremes are canoe, tent, and car camping. Canoe camping offers remoteness with the convenience of being able to effortlessly lug along goodies. Most of us get a kick out of tent camping or car camping, where we can spend the evening around a campfire and sleep under the stars but don't have to leave our sodas and steaks at home.

If you take a few simple precautions, camping during pregnancy will be safe and fun—even if it's your first time sleeping in the woods. Plus, all the preparations you need to make for camping during pregnancy will give you practice for getting out in the wilderness with your baby. For children, camping provides both the ultimate adventure and a supreme education.

No matter how you enjoy the outdoors while camping, whether hiking, sunbathing, bird watching, fishing, splashing around in the creek, or simply hanging around camp, you'll get a real break from your daily grind. And that's exactly what you may need during pregnancy—a little peace and quiet, and a lot of wilderness.

RISK ASSESSMENT BY TRIMESTER

    1ST TRIMESTER: LOW
    2ND TRIMESTER: LOW
    3RD TRIMESTER: MEDIUM

Staying Healthy Each Trimester

1ST TRIMESTER | RISK: LOW

Even if you are only an occasional camper, you can really enjoy being out in the woods during pregnancy—especially during your first trimester. Camping is a great way to experience the wilderness without exerting yourself too much. And that's just perfect this trimester, when your energy level may be low.

Before you head out, honestly assess your needs and concerns. It is common to feel more protective of your safety during pregnancy. After all, your baby is growing inside you. If sleeping outdoors makes you nervous, think about bringing an RV or camper van—even if you're a master tent camper. If you have to urinate several times a night, keep slippers and a flashlight handy and choose a site close to the restroom. If your back has been bothering you, try a self-inflating sleeping pad that offers good support. If nausea has been a problem, bring along your favorite crackers and try sucking on ginger candy to help with carsickness.

Second, assess your risks. Take into account the weather, the altitude gain, the campsite resources, and your needs. Always camp with a reliable friend. And estimate your stamina conservatively. Then make a cautious plan. If you are in terrific shape and are an experienced backpacker, you might try hiking in to a remote site this trimester. Or try canoeing in to camp along a river or lake where you don't have to carry your gear. Most campgrounds have a few walk-in sites that feel attractively remote, but are less than a mile from the car.

This trimester, you can take the same kinds of camping trips you have enjoyed before. Tent, camper, and RV camping should be a piece of cake. Just pay particular attention to clean water and toilet access. If you're feeling more adventurous still, a two- or three-day backpacking trip is safe as long as you are an experienced backpacker. Since you'll feel exhausted more quickly, however, stay away from the hard-core adventures like snow camping, extended backpacking, or trips that require carrying heavy gear.

camping

Spending a couple of days outdoors could help you overcome distressing first-trimester mood swings and insomnia. Relaxing and getting away from your daily stresses may help a lot. Just being active around camp will give you enough of a workout to get your appetite up and help you sleep better. Plus, fresh air can do wonders for nausea.

2ND TRIMESTER | RISK: LOW

Your growing belly shouldn't get in the way of your enjoying a great camping trip with your family and friends this trimester. And you probably have the appetite and extra energy to really get a kick out of all the fun around camp and the surrounding wilderness.

If you are longing to get away from it all for weekend and need to get a little wilderness back in your life, go camping. You'll notice that your sleeping pad isn't as kind to your back as your bed, crouching over a toilet isn't as easy when you're front-heavy, and the cold showers (or no showers) may even make your fetus kick, but you'll feel revitalized and refreshed anyway. Throw in some of your favorite outdoor activities while you're out there or just stretch out on your sleeping pad and watch the clouds. Camping is a great way to get back in touch with yourself—and with the remarkable natural process your body is going through.

To protect your back and to stick closer to help, stay away from challenging overnight backpacking trips where you have to carry all your gear and water in to a remote camp. And never camp alone. Instead, indulge in some safe car or tent camping. A camper or a good tent offers reassuring protection from the elements, especially if the weather turns.

When packing for a camping trip this trimester, don't hesitate to bring a few extras: snacks, a comfortable, thick sleeping pad, and cozy clothes for cool evenings. Don't forget sunscreen, pregnancy-safe mosquito repellent, and supportive shoes. Get some help carrying the gear, though, since lugging large coolers and heavy tents yourself can injure your back.

If you've been pretty active this trimester, camping opens up a world of possible activities, from kayaking to making s'mores to exploring new trails. If you haven't managed to get out of the house much yet, camping may help revitalize your love of the outdoors and help you get in better shape for your third trimester and delivery.

In my fourth month, I gamely planned a camping trip to Yellowstone and Glacier national parks with my husband. Our meandering road trip would culminate in four days in the wilderness—well, in a campground with running water and toilets, in the wilderness.

While packing my gear as I had done a hundred times before, I was suddenly overcome by strange thoughts. Would I be comfortable enough on my Thermarest? Would I be able to get out of the tent fast enough to pee in the middle of the night? Could campfire smoke harm the baby? What about grizzlies?!

I began to recognize an unusual and startling emotion: fear. Never before had I been anxious when going camping. The idea of seeing bears in the wilderness normally excited me—instead of filling me with trepidation. I wondered, was this my protective maternal instinct or just crazy hormones?

But my husband's enthusiasm was contagious and this was our vacation, after all. Binoculars in hand, I was ready to see some wildlife— from a safe distance. Our car was stuffed, since we brought along some things we wouldn't normally have worried about, like a water filter, extra pillows, extra sleeping pads, and slip-on shoes for nighttime emergencies. And our focus was a little different than usual: we didn't do a monster hike. Instead, we took a creekside trail near camp and spent hours birdwatching. The scenery was spectacular and the campfire dinner as cozy and satisfying as always. It was exactly the break we both needed.

The trip turned out fine—no bears attacked and I became a pro at the midnight quick exit from the tent (even in the rain). And in the spirit of compromise and comfort, we spent one night in a hotel.

—Jennifer, Olympia, Washington

camping

Unless you are really active, you probably won't feel like venturing too far from the house this trimester, let alone into the wilderness to spend the night. And that's good thinking. Your belly and tender back will make sleeping on the ground—not to mention getting up and down—less than comfortable. Plus, you'll have to watch out for early signs of labor, like back pain with tension across your belly, that mean that you need to stick close to help—and, ideally, close to your own doctor.

Camping is medium-risk activity this trimester because you may go into labor—preterm or on time—and need urgent medical attention. If you insist on spending the night in the wilderness, always have someone responsible with you and look for camping sites within an hour of a metropolitan-area hospital. You'll be surprised at how many attractive options there are, even near home.

Other than proximity to help, your primary concern will be comfort. Late in pregnancy, a sleeping bag can feel quite constraining, especially when you sleep on your side (as you should be). One solution is to zip together two bags. Or look into renting a camper with beds fitted with standard linens. As throughout pregnancy, ensure that you have access to plenty of potable water. Also, take time to acclimatize before sleeping at high altitude (you should sleep below eight thousand feet) since you are more susceptible to altitude illness, especially if you are coming from sea level.

Once you're situated at the campsite, you'll have a lot of fun. Of course, you may not be up for a great deal of mountaineering and swimming, but you can take some walks around the campground, enjoy the rowdy camp spirit, and share in the fun from a comfortable seat nearby.

Don't panic if you feel a few contractions—this is normal. These Braxton Hicks contractions and should go away as soon as you sit down and rest for a few minutes. They will *not* harm your baby and do not mean you automatically need to head home at the speed of light. Just take it easy and get someone else to cook or set up camp until the contractions go away.

Equipment Considerations

All of us have camping rituals that make us really savor the camping experience and treasure it like no other occasion. Everyone has their own definition of *essential* gear for their camping trip. It may include a set of spices for seasoning the camp food, a guitar, an old multipurpose bandanna, woolly moccasins, or a portable espresso maker. During pregnancy, you'll discover a few more essentials, like a good flashlight and convenient flip-flops.

Drinking water is at the top of the list. You'll need to bring a specialized water filter or a pot for boiling water to make it potable, just in case no safe water can be found. Identifying safe water in the woods can be tricky, but I use this rule of thumb: if the park service has labeled a fountain "potable water," you can drink it. If not, you need to assume it is not safe. This doesn't mean that brushing your teeth with stream water will harm your baby, but it could make you sick to your stomach and pretty dehydrated as a result of vomiting and diarrhea.

If you happen to be looking for new gear, you'll be lucky enough to be able to take your pregnancy into consideration when choosing equipment. Make sure you get in there and test everything. I mean it: crawl in the bag and the tent and move around to see how they feel. Will that mummy bag be roomy enough for a big belly? Does the tent have enough space for you to comfortably change clothes? Does your backpack distribute the load on your hips so that your back is protected? Will these hiking shoes be easy to put on and take off when you can't bend over so easily? Keep in mind that you're also buying gear to last many years and it should meet your longterm needs as well.

You don't need fancy gear to have a good time. Just make sure you pack warm layers and are prepared for unexpected weather changes. Don't get caught in a freak summer hailstorm without raingear (although in that event you might decide to bundle up and enjoy a game of cards in the tent).

Preparing for Difficult Situations

Depending on where you go camping, some conditions may make the excursion more challenging and potentially hazardous to your pregnancy. Think about your site and plan before heading out. Do you have to hike in to the camp or can you drive right up to it? Obviously, the easier the access, the safer the site. What kind of terrain is around the campsite? If it is groomed and well maintained, you are less likely to risk falling—especially important when you're making your way to the restroom in the dark. Is there flat space for a tent or sleeping bags? Sleeping well during pregnancy is important, especially if you have been active all day.

camping

How far is the nearest hospital? I recommend being within an hour's drive—tent-to-door—of a hospital with some obstetric capacity. The clinic in the park or in a nearby small town will probably not be open at night or even on weekends, but it may have a doctor on call, so jot down the number. Also check the cell phone coverage so you can get help immediately if you need it.

Are there restrooms and water fountains with drinkable water? Is there a park ranger who patrols the area? Is there shade? At what altitude is the campsite? Are the insects out and are there any local insect-borne diseases, like Lyme disease, you should protect yourself against? A good insect repellent is all you need. What about bigger pests, like raccoons or bears? Just follow the park ranger's instructions for storing your food (some campsites have bear-proof containers) and you shouldn't have any furry visitors at night. Here's a very important tip: Don't keep your food in your tent with you.

Once you've answered these questions, you will be well prepared to head out on a terrific camping trip and handle unexpected hassles along the way.

Planning Pointers for Pregnancy

1 Choose a well-maintained campground. A campground within a state or national park should have some of the amenities that make camping easier, like drinking water, picnic tables, restrooms with toilet paper, shade, and groomed campsites. You may also have car access directly to the campsite or hookups for electricity and RV sewer systems. Just call ahead of time and ask.

2 Bring comfortable gear. Bring shoes that give good arch and ankle support for daytime and a pair of slip-ons and a flashlight for trips to the bathroom at night. Bring a sleeping bag that will keep you warm enough—an all-season bag may be more comfortable than your thin summer bag. Don't forget a sleeping pad; I recommend a self-inflating pad to protect your tender back.

3 Pack layers. Only bring cozy clothing, and layers of it. You may end up wearing two sets of long underwear, two pairs of socks, a vest, a sweater, and a sweat-shirt—all at once. Who cares? Only the birds are watching. Check weather reports for local highs and lows so you can pack accordingly.

4 Skip the backpack. Unless you are a dedicated backpacker and you just can't stay off the trails (during your first trimester only), try car camping instead. You'll be closer to help if you need it and you'll be able to carry some goodies that will make camping truly relaxing, like your favorite pillow and the ingredients for a hearty meal. If you do backpack in to camp, carry as little weight as possible, don't get too remote (cell phone access is a plus).

5 Make sure you have plenty of drinking water. Your most likely risk is simply getting too dehydrated on the trail and overexerting yourself. Taking it easy is good for you and your developing baby.

6 Camp with friends and family. Camping is a social occasion. And that's part of what makes it safe during pregnancy. Get help carrying gear and always let someone know where you are going and when you plan to return—even if you're only going for a stroll around camp.

7 Avoid the heat. Avoid camping on very hot or humid days, when you may overheat. The inside of your tent can become an oven, so pick a site with shade and air out your tent in the evening before turning in.

8 Know how to get help. Take a look at the map to locate the nearest town and hospital before choosing your campsite and check with your cell phone company to see if it offers service in that area. Check in with the park ranger or camp resident when you get to camp.

9 Soak in the wilderness. Camping is your chance to get away from it all and reset your priorities. When you're living outside, even for a couple of days, you'll take time to find that bird that's been singing its heart out all morning. When was the last time you watched the moon rise? Take a deep breath—and take some of that wilderness back home with you. It will nourish you throughout the rest of your pregnancy.

mountain biking

If you are an experienced mountain biker, off-road riding is a fun way to blow off some steam. Admit it: you do it for the adrenaline. No doubt you savor the rush of tackling a rugged single-track uphill trail and challenging yourself on the technical hops on the way down. For most mountain biking enthusiasts, the fun is in the hair-raising danger and sheer speed—and the natural beauty. You probably pick your trails for the number of stream crossings, remoteness, and lack of other bikers and hikers to get in the way of your riding.

There is a tamer version of mountain biking, however: that of groomed dirt and the serenely winding path. This is the ride I encourage you to look for during pregnancy. You just don't want to risk a broken wrist or a cracked collarbone (one of the most common mountain biking injuries) while your body is already coping with the enormous changes of pregnancy. Choose safer trails and avoid obstacles so that you can ride without fear. And rule out mountain biking completely after your first trimester, when your growing fetus is vulnerable to injury too.

Mountain biking can be just as much about the awesome surroundings—the tranquility of a shaded stream or the sudden sun in a meadow—as the exhilaration of the ride. A gentler, graded ride in pretty country will give you an excellent workout without wearing you out—or throwing you over the handlebars.

Understandably, you are likely to be cautious about getting on a bike, let alone going off-road, during pregnancy. Follow your instincts: if you are nervous on a bike, just stick to a comfortable hike instead. Mountain biking requires a high level of fitness, skill, confidence, and comfort with your brakes, gears, and toe clips. Not there yet? Don't worry; you have lots of other attractive options.

If you don't bike off road very often, stay on level paths as much as possible. Dirt or gravel service roads or fire roads in parks (they are usually off limits to cars) are an excellent way to get away from traffic and hikers and get deep into some stunning scenery. Or look for a ridge trail that bypasses the switchbacks coming up the mountain and the single track on the descent. Whether you explore familiar local trails or head out for a weekend of mountain biking at a ski resort during the off-season (no, you won't be screaming straight down the downhill course), you'll be able to find plenty of great, safe rides.

mountain biking

If you are an avid mountain biker and are in good shape, there is little reason to stay off the trails during your first trimester. Riding a bike is easier on your joints than hiking (especially if you're tackling some hills), but it's tough on your muscles, so it's good aerobic exercise. I guarantee you'll feel your heart pumping—even more so because you are pregnant. Just pick your trails wisely, stay cool, and bike with someone who will look out for you. I mean this literally: having a buddy riding ahead of you and calling out upcoming obstacles will help you slow down and ride defensively. Biking with a group can be fun, as long as you aren't racing and you can stick with bikers below your usual level (this is no time to show off). Stopping to chat will give you a chance to drink up and avoid overexertion. If you feel unwell, stop, rest, and take the easy way back.

Like any good exercise, mountain biking is healthiest if it's part of a regular exercise program. Since, if you're like most people, you'll only mountain bike sporadically—a weekend here, an afternoon there—you should take up some other activities to keep up your stamina and maintain your strength and flexibility. Not only will a regular workout (whether it is road biking, hiking, or swimming) be good for your mountain biking, it's very good for the health of your fetus. If you do something active for at least half an hour three times a week (including your mountain biking), you'll notice that you have more energy, a better appetite, improved sleep, and a good attitude. Plus, you'll have established good exercise habits for the rest of your pregnancy.

RISK ASSESSMENT BY TRIMESTER

1ST TRIMESTER: MEDIUM
2ND TRIMESTER: HIGH
3RD TRIMESTER: HIGH

Staying Healthy Each Trimester

1ST TRIMESTER | RISK: MEDIUM

If you're tempted to hit the trails this trimester and are a confident mountain biker, go for it. There is nothing like a good ride to make you feel strong and independent—and give you back some of the old "you" you may be missing.

"Six years before my first pregnancy, I entered the expert class of mountain bike racing and fantasized about trying my hand at pro racing. It seems hard to believe now, but I actually postponed pregnancy because I knew it would interfere with my biking. And of course it did. Even when I forgot about the pregnancy for a few instants of sheer riding bliss, one of my mates would swing by with a fruit roll or point out an upcoming rock and I'd remember that everyone else remembered. And that support felt good.

I abandoned my regular training regimen and went biking strictly for fun. To be honest, I was too exhausted most of the time to do anything regularly, although I did wheel out the bike often to run errands.

Where and how I biked totally changed. I wasn't really afraid of falling, but I had developed a deep sense of caution and awareness of my body. Basically, I took it slow. Annoyingly, the mantra "I think I can, I think I can" accompanied me on many uphills. Contrary to every mountain biking instinct in my body, I was downright relieved to find flat trails with a view—and bushes, since I had to stop every few miles to pee.

We found a bunch of service roads through the nearby park system that were blocked off to cars and shunned by hikers seeking trails, and just perfect for biking. I switched to a taller tourist stem as my belly got bigger and just kept cruising until the baby was born. As soon as we could take our little one in the bike trailer, we went back to these roads—not too bumpy to wake a two-month-old and not too steep to wear out an ex-expert-biker mama.

—Mina, Burlington, Vermont"

mountain biking

Just let caution guide you so that you don't fall—and you don't "bonk." "Bonking" is how mountain bikers describe everything from dizziness to dehydration and overheating to headaches. And you don't want any of these maladies to happen to you—especially when you're pregnant, because they are not good for your fetus, either. And since your body is in overdrive anyway, you are more vulnerable to these problems. That is why I consider mountain biking somewhat risky even this early in pregnancy. Any endurance sport, particularly one like trail riding that pushes you hard and exposes you to the elements, can sap your energy.

The key to preventing overheating and overexertion, or bonking, on the trail is good preparation. First, you need a lot of water. Hit the trail with at least a liter of water for every hour you plan to exercise. You don't even have to stop biking to hydrate—just grab the bottle off the bike and squirt it into your mouth. Second, keep high-protein snacks within reach. Third, take breaks to chat and chew.

Most important, plan conservative rides. This means shorter and easier. It doesn't mean less beautiful or less fun. I recommend a *maximum* ride of an hour, including breaks, warm-up, and cooldown. Most women say they are comfortable biking about half the distance they used to before pregnancy. The distance you cover on your ride will depend on the trail, the elevation change, and your level of fitness. For a moderate one-hour ride, five miles is a reasonable goal.

If you make mountain biking a part of a regular exercise program this trimester, you'll not only enjoy your outdoors time but also stay fit, have less nausea, and enjoy a better appetite. Plus, doing something you really love will inspire you to stay active during pregnancy.

2ND TRIMESTER | RISK: HIGH

If you've hammered downhill before, the wind whipping past your ears, you know the risks of mountain biking. Gripping the edge of a cliff, skidding through dust, and splashing across moving water, you're on the verge of falling—and it gives you a rush. But as your belly grows and your developing baby becomes more exposed to possible injury, it's just not worth it.

After about twelve weeks of gestation, your uterus protrudes into your abdominal cavity, beyond the solid protection of your pubic bone, where it can be struck directly in a fall: handlebars to belly, for example. Not only that, but the growing uterus is less stabilized and even a sudden stop can seriously harm the placenta. For these reasons, off-road biking is far too risky after your first trimester. If you are eager to stay in the saddle this trimester, try biking flat, groomed paths with little traffic—and no obstacles.

3RD TRIMESTER | RISK: HIGH

I doubt you'll even consider hopping on a bicycle this trimester, unless it's a cruiser with wide wheels and a comfy seat, or a stationary reclining model that allows plenty of room for your belly and doesn't require any balance. And that's how it should be. As you'd expect, your risk of falling and endangering your pregnancy is greatest during your third trimester. Mountain biking, with its unpredictable terrain, sudden turns, high level of physical exertion, and likelihood of falls, is simply not a good idea.

That doesn't mean you have to stay inside: getting outdoors will help relieve stress, pass the time, and keep you fit for delivery. Try hiking some of the trails you have biked (just watch out for reckless bikers!). If you can't stay away from biking and you are an experienced biker, take your mountain bike on bike *paths*—not trails. Because the frame is more upright and the handlebars higher than a regular road bike, you may find that a mountain bike is really comfortable, even late in pregnancy, as long as you are on level, paved trails.

Warming Up

Before you hit the trail, take five minutes to warm up by biking a flat area (the trailhead parking lot) or walking around. Then do some dynamic stretches (see chapter 6), targeting your legs, calves, arms, and back, to prevent injuries and soreness. You'll find that activating your arms and back helps you maintain good posture while riding so you don't get a sore back.

Mountain Biking Technique for Pregnancy

During pregnancy—for your and your fetus's sake—you need to ride efficiently, so you don't get worn out and overheated. Also, your joints are somewhat relaxed now, so you want to treat them with care. Use the techniques below to make your riding safer and more comfortable during pregnancy.

mountain biking

Good biking posture will protect your delicate knee and hip joints. When you pedal, keep your knees together so that you are using your quadriceps (the muscles at the front of your thighs) and your abdominals to power yourself. Instead of stomping on the pedals—which is not good for your knees—push and pull the pedals around in a complete rotation so both feet are working for you all the time. Stay away from toe clips after your first trimester, because they could increase your chances of being inextricably attached to the pedals and falling.

Keep up a steady rhythm of pedaling by changing gears and adjusting your pace rather than fervently pedaling in bursts followed by panting, speechlessness, and exhaustion. Slow and steady wins the race.

Cooling Down

When you are exhilarated and exhausted at the end of a ride, it's tempting to gather around the drinking fountain to talk about the ride, forgetting to cool down. But you'll regret it later. Cooling down is all about preventing soreness. Five minutes of walking around or biking leisurely will also help your blood circulate and maintain healthy blood flow to your fetus. Just walk in circles around the drinking fountain if you have to so you can still participate in the conversation. Mountain biking is very tough on your legs—you can already feel *that*—and on your arms and back. Try some pregnancy-safe stretches while your muscles are still warm to relax them and keep them flexible.

Equipment Considerations

You must have a good helmet to mountain bike. There are no two ways about it: no helmet, no ride. If you don't already have a trusted and undamaged helmet, buy one that is comfortable and fits like a glove. It shouldn't be perched on the back of your head like a beret and shouldn't move when you shake your head. It should fit snugly about an inch above your eyebrows. The strap should be snug enough around your chin that you can't slip a finger in or even chew with your helmet on. You just don't want that helmet flying off when you spill.

Customizing your equipment can help you be a better and more comfortable rider. Adjust your seat height and position so you have the maximum leverage with each stroke—which means more power. If you sit on the seat with one foot flat on a pedal at the bottom of its rotation, your leg should be almost completely straight, not locked. With the proper seat height, you'll protect your back and you'll be less sore overall at the end of the day. And when you're pregnant, the last thing you need is more achiness in your back

You may find that your crotch gets pretty sore when you ride. This is because pregnancy increases the blood flow to the genital area, making it more sensitive. The solution is to wear padded bike shorts, sit on a molded seat, and take frequent breaks to stretch and shake it up. You may not feel like putting on those tight shorts while you're gaining all this (healthy) weight, but it's worth it. Bike shorts and pants have a special gel crotch and they are more comfortable than they look. Plus, they stretch right over your growing belly, don't get all bunched up, and don't cause chafing. And they don't get snagged on the saddle. You can also check out saddles built for women, which are somewhat shorter and wider than the one you probably have on your bike.

Make sure you have the equipment to carry the trail essentials: full water bottles, snacks, and a bike lock (just in case you decide to hike instead). This includes a comfortable day or hydration backpack, at least one bottle holder, and a repair-kit and pump in case a rock blows your tire.

Preparing for Difficult Situations

You'll have a great bike ride if you're confident about your skills and know what to expect along the way. No matter where you bike, you'll need to think carefully about things that will make the ride especially challenging, like the length, intensity, terrain, remoteness, and rescue accessibility of the trail. Even if you are biking in a local park, you need to know the answers to the following questions: Are there shortcuts I could take if I needed to? Is the return ride uphill? Is there a lot of bike, horse, or hiker traffic? Is the trail well maintained? Are there restrooms and water fountains? Is there a park ranger who patrols the area? Are there muddy, rocky, or underwater parts of the trail? Is there shade? With these answers, you'll be sure you'll back safe and sound.

If you are going to a state park, national forest, or an off-season ski resort to bike, you are guaranteed to catch some awe-inspiring scenery and uninterrupted riding. Just watch out for the altitude (stay below eight thousand feet if you're coming from sea level), sudden weather changes, unsafe water, and insects. With some simple preparation, you'll be in good shape.

Planning Pointers for Pregnancy

1 Bike with confidence. In your first trimester, if mountain biking will make your week, go for it! Get dirty and find yourself some solitude and a thrill or two. Stick to paths where you are very comfortable and you can ride without fear. This is no time for daredevil stunts or grueling mega-rides. Stick to groomed or paved paths if you're inexperienced, or if you're past your first trimester.

2 Choose trails for safety. Enjoy a conservative ride. This means choosing sweeping cross-country trails rather than single-track switchbacks. Look for dirt service roads, ridge trails, and meandering creekside paths that offer fantastic scenery—without the sweat-drenched climbs and hair-raising descents.

3 Prevent bonking. Mountain biking can easily sap your energy and cause dehydration and overheating, otherwise known as "bonking." Listen to your body so that you can anticipate your needs, pace yourself, and rest *before* you feel unwell. Plan to go at a slower pace, travel a shorter distance, take more breaks, and be flexible about when you turn back.

4 Helmet. Helmet. Helmet. Don't even think about riding without it.

5 Ride with friends. Mountain biking with friends or a club is especially fun, especially if it ends in a swim in the ocean or a picnic. Plus, you'll be more likely to stop, chat, and keep your energy up, and you'll have help—just in case.

6 Drink up. Even in cool weather, you lose tons of water when biking. Make sure you are carrying plenty of water and keep drinking on the trail.

7 Pace yourself. You need to stay cool, so don't wear yourself out on a climb. It's okay to just get off and walk up. Try to maintain a steady pace by switching gears and taking frequent breaks.

8 Warm up and cool down. You'll be tempted to jump right on the bike as soon as you take it off the rack, but it's a lot healthier for you—and your baby—to warm up first. Focus on your legs, but don't forget your arms and back, which support your posture on the bike. Cooling down is important for preventing soreness and maintaining healthy blood flow to your fetus.

9 Look around. If you're just focused on the patch of dirt a few feet ahead of your front wheel, it's easy to miss the dramatic beauty all around you. Since you're riding slower now, you'll be able to appreciate some of the scenery you may have whizzed right by a few months ago.

rock climbing

Rock climbing requires strength, agility, and will power. It is an endurance sport with an adrenaline edge. And the rewards are high—quite literally. Women are taking up rock climbing because it offers great personal satisfaction and also calls for strong teamwork. Working toward a summit several hundred—or several thousand—feet off terra firma is truly a test of one's abilities; a test best postponed until after pregnancy.

Being far off the ground is the primarily reason that traditional and sport climbing is hazardous. For one, a lead fall could be catastrophic for your pregnancy. Although the fetus is well protected behind the pubic bone in the first trimester, your suffering a serious injury, such as a pelvic fracture or head injury, would endanger your ability to carry the pregnancy. Second, most day climbs, even with a partner providing good belay support, do not allow you to take extended, comfortable breaks. Although early in pregnancy your growing uterus may not interfere with your pushing hard on a vertical climb, your fatigue and nausea will slow you down. The need to take regular breaks should keep you closer to level ground.

Pregnancy loosens your ligaments, increasing your chances of straining a joint with reaching and pumping to maintain stability. Elbow and finger injuries are also a risk, especially if you are not able to back off and stretch regularly. As the pregnancy progresses, your center of gravity changes, altering your balance on the rock and increasing your chances of injury. And as the uterus grows into the abdomen by your third month, your fetus becomes especially vulnerable. Other than rock (or object) falls and taking a lead fall, harness straps across the abdomen are another source of direct trauma to the uterus. Keep in mind that even hard jumps can traumatize the delicate placenta, causing an abruption (tearing the placenta from the uterine wall).

The safest way to approach rocks during early pregnancy is with the aim to improve your technique and balance and stick closer to the ground. All you need are rock shoes and chalk. Bouldering offers its own challenges: perfecting difficult moves, improving your traversing skill, and learning to link moves without gaining height. You can enjoy bouldering without ropes, but if you're set on mastering rope technique close to ground, use a "top rope" technique (the rope runs from the climber up through a secure anchor at the top of a rock and back down to the belayer), which is more secure. Also, note that during pregnancy the harness will make your engorged crotch especially sore. Sticking near ground will allow you to stow away that harness until after delivery (you'll probably feel up to getting vertical again within a few weeks of having that baby).

When bouldering, your risk of falling badly is much less, especially if you take along a partner to spot you; a spotter should stand behind you and protect your back and head from hitting anything if you fall. Another safety option is a bouldering pad, which gets positioned under the crux, or the most difficult portion of the bouldering route. Best of all, you can hop down to the ground regularly and take a breather—for hydration, stretching, and a snack—and get some perspective on your route.

Later in pregnancy, gain vertical distance on a scenic hiking trail. You'll still get a great workout and get outdoors, but your focus will be on maintaining your mental, rather than physical, balance. Several pregnancy-safe activities, like swimming and hiking, help build strength and flexibility in the muscles you need for climbing and prepare you well for the rest of pregnancy. Your stamina and motivation to get outdoors will help you stay active and fit for your next climbing session—and for the endurance test of delivery.

RISK ASSESSMENT BY TRIMESTER

1ST TRIMESTER: HIGH
2ND TRIMESTER: HIGH
3RD TRIMESTER: HIGH

mountaineering

There is something addictive about climbing high into the sky—it must be the adventure and the adrenaline rush—and it may cloud your ability to reason when it comes to deciding whether to head out during pregnancy.

The fact is that high-altitude exposure is not safe for your developing baby. Yes, people live at high altitude and have healthy babies—in the Andes and even in the Rockies. But living at high altitude causes the body to make countless subtle adjustments over a period of years to remain healthy and robust. Visiting a high-altitude location, even if you're in terrific shape, doesn't come with these advantages. Doing intense exercise at high altitude, such as mountaineering, is even tougher on the body. The negative effects of high altitude on pregnancy, especially over eight thousand feet, are well documented. You are more vulnerable to altitude illness during pregnancy and are susceptible to becoming ill even at lower altitudes if you are coming from near sea level.

The rules are simple: If you live at a lower altitude, your trail should stay below six thousand feet. Brief passes to eight thousand feet should be safe, if you are well acclimatized, or accustomed to the decreased oxygen level. It may take a few days to get used to the altitude, even when you are simply hanging around camp. Look out for the headache, nausea, and fatigue that accompany mild altitude illness. These are signals that you and your fetus are not getting an ideal oxygen supply. Rest, hydrate well, and descend if the symptoms don't resolve to protect your and your fetus's health.

No ropes, no picks, and no crampons. Using this gear means hard terrain, a risky climb, and extreme conditions. Falls on wilderness trails are very dangerous for anyone because rescue is so difficult and can take days to arrange. It's just not worth the risk during pregnancy.

This is not to say that you have to quit "peak bagging" altogether during pregnancy. If it's a view or the highest point around you're aiming for, most are well within reach during pregnancy. For example, common goals for people who want to climb everything in sight include New Hampshire's forty-eight four-thousand-foot peaks and the Adirondacks' forty-six four-thousand-footers.

If you're a mountaineer, you must already be in great shape and have a driving passion for the outdoors, which will keep you active—and very healthy—throughout pregnancy. You have lots of options. To glimpse wildlife, try paddling a nearby river instead. To get away from it all, try snowshoeing. To catch wild-flowers in bloom, try hiking a lower elevation trail—you'll see more color well below the tree line anyway!

If you're an avid hiker and backpacker, take a look at the tips in the Hiking section for how to stay safe and healthy on the trail. If you want that mountain climbing experience without having to carry a lot of gear and overexert your-self, look for remote lodges that offer overnight accommodation and meals. Northwest Montana's Glacier National Park, Tennessee and North Carolina's Great Smoky Mountains National Park, and New Hampshire's White Mountains offer a few good options. You can enjoy the satisfaction of reaching your climb-ing goal, watch the wildlife during peak hours at dusk and dawn, drink lemonade by moonlight, and sigh as you lie your tired body down on a soft bed. Not bad for a compromise, eh?

Mountaineering is for experts. You need courage, strength, and endurance to handle the conditions on a mountain. Altitude illness, heat exhaustion, cold exposure, and even a sprained ankle can become life threatening if you are far from help, your judgment is affected, or the weather changes. You are more vul-nerable to these threats during pregnancy.

I recommend sticking closer to help—and weather forecasts—in places where the scenery is no less breathtaking. A serene hike through rolling hills will connect you to the awe-inspiring changes within your own body—and you may find there is more natural beauty *inside* than you expected.

RISK ASSESSMENT BY TRIMESTER

1ST TRIMESTER: HIGH

2ND TRIMESTER: HIGH

3RD TRIMESTER: HIGH

horseback riding

Horseback riding is an exhilarating sport that requires flexibility, balance, and an intimate relationship with a large and powerful animal. Even the most cherished and trusted horse can be unpredictable when startled or irritated. Shying, bucking, balking, and rearing are among its forms of communication. Although you may be able to control and direct a well-behaved horse, a whole host of unexpected factors, such as insect bites, snakes, heat, illness, bad manners, hormones, and even plain moodiness can make the horse wild and put you at its mercy. I don't just mean a temperamental nip in the seat of your pants with its teeth. Remember, your horse is an athlete too: sleek, muscular, alert, and raring to go.

Horseback riding is a very risky activity during pregnancy, because you are entirely dependent on the horse's good behavior. If it starts galloping for whatever reason and won't stop, you have no escape. Subtle changes in your weight and center of gravity also affect how you ride, how your balance changes with the horse's gait, and how the horse responds to you. If you lose your balance or your saddle slips, you are more likely to fall and hurt yourself. The distance, the speed, the hardness of the ground, and the likely tangles with stirrups add to this risk.

The rhythm of the horse's gait, while it can feel soothing, is physically traumatic for your pregnant body. That achy crotch following a horseback ride is even worse when that area receives an increased blood flow, making you more sensitive and more bruised. The bouncing and jarring of riding a horse also strains your relaxed pelvic ligaments and jostles the growing uterus. You can even endure damage to your pubic bone and endanger your pregnancy.

Even if you are a true cowgirl with a trusty steed and can somehow guarantee walking and trotting only and no falls—if that were possible—don't even consider riding after your first trimester. After twelve weeks, the risk of serious injury to your growing fetus becomes far greater because the uterus is less protected by the public bone. Rough terrain and aggressive riding, such as cantering, galloping, and jumping, are obviously off-limits too throughout the entire pregnancy.

I don't mean to say that you need to stay away from the horse and stable you love so dearly. Caring for horses during pregnancy is safe—as long as you know what you're doing and someone else is exercising them. If you're a dedicated rider, you'll find it difficult to stay out of the stable for that long anyway.

Just the warm, musty smell of hay and the camaraderie of the barn provide a healthy break from the rest of your daily responsibilities. Your horse needs your care and attention as much as you need that soft touch. Believe it or not, grooming your own horse is a great way to stay fit. Rubbing down, sponging, and currycombing require patience and upper-body strength and give you a good workout.

Walking around the stable grounds while distributing oats, hiking familiar riding trails, and throwing a tattered ball to the barn dog are great exercise during pregnancy. You can also learn a lot by watching other experts ride and observing lessons.

Let common sense guide you around the stable. Steer clear of irritable horses. Use your legs, not your back, when lifting oats or gear and get help when you need to move anything over twenty-five pounds. You'll need to stay away from riding, but you can get out to the stable as often as you like—just don't forget to bring alfalfa.

If you were a regular rider and have good technique, your well toned back and leg muscles and excellent posture will pay off during pregnancy. You'll probably have fewer aches and pains as your belly grows—and you'll still have your passion for getting outdoors and feeling the wind in your hair. Just find safer options for feeding this passion, such as hiking, biking, and camping.

RISK ASSESSMENT BY TRIMESTER

1ST TRIMESTER: HIGH
2ND TRIMESTER: HIGH
3RD TRIMESTER: HIGH

chapter

10

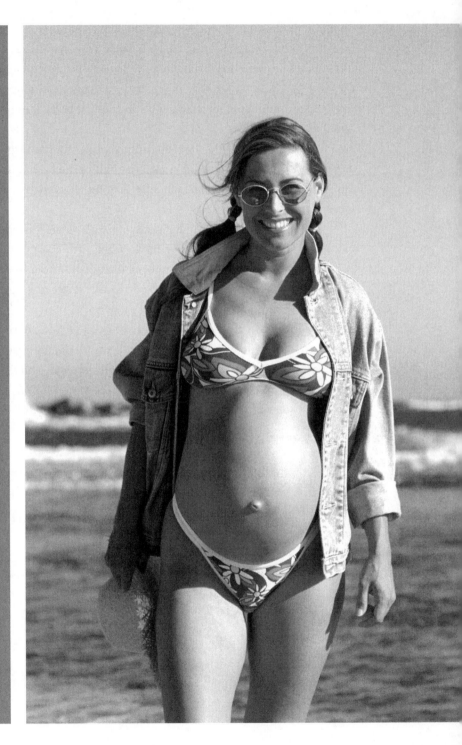

Staying Active on the Water

There is a feeling of magic that accompanies being in water during pregnancy. The weightlessness of simply floating can take you out of your growing, unwieldy body—at least for a few minutes. For this reason, swimming is one of the most popular activities during pregnancy. There's a lot of room for adventure beyond the prenatal swim session at the local gym, however. Water sports like snorkeling and kayaking are excellent options when you're expecting.

Exercising in water has enormous benefits for pregnant women: it's an excellent cardiovascular workout; it reduces ankle swelling; and it keeps you cool even as you work all your muscles. There aren't a lot of sports that actually improve with pregnancy, but some water sports do. Some women find that their lower center of gravity and increased joint flexibility improve their paddling posture and efficiency, for example.

If you haven't been very active before pregnancy and are ready to get going, water activities like swimming or canoeing are great places to start because they are easy on your pregnant body. If you are a water mama who's tempted to water ski, windsurf, or surf through pregnancy, you should carefully consider your risks before hitting the waves. No matter what, get wet. It's healthy for you and your fetus and it's a special way to commune with the swimmer inside your own watery womb.

swimming

Swimming is a great way to get off your feet and still get some good exercise. Playing in the water is refreshing and relaxing. Swimming provides an excellent aerobic workout but is gentle on the joints, especially knees and hips. The buoyancy of the water supports your body (you feel almost weightless) while offering resistance for your muscles so that you build strength and stamina.

Did I say *weightless*? Yes, swimming is such a popular activity during pregnancy because you can float. It just feels wonderful to have that weight lifted off your tired back and legs—especially later in pregnancy when other exercises may really wear you out. Unlike most other exercise, swimming tones your entire body, including the vital muscles that support you during pregnancy: your legs, back, and abdominals. Even if you are not a very strong swimmer, you can keep your feet on the bottom or dog-paddle and still get a good workout. If you propel yourself through the water, whether you are swimming the breaststroke, gripping a kickboard, cruising on your back, or even running, you'll get your heart rate up too and be in better shape for delivery.

Water exercise has several unique properties that make it particularly safe during pregnancy. One is that you can't really *fall* and hurt yourself—the water supports you. Your buoyancy helps prevent injuries, as long as you are a confident swimmer or stay in shallow water. Jumping and diving are not a good idea, however, because you can hurt your belly, and water can be forced up into your vagina, possibly causing an infection. And, stay away from contact sports in the water, like water polo, where you could be hit directly in the belly or held underwater. Another benefit of swimming is that water conducts heat away from your body twenty-five times more efficiently than air does, keeping you cool and protecting your fetus from overheating. Water activities are particularly useful during your first trimester when overheating is a risk and could affect your fetus's development.

Another perk of water activities during pregnancy is that simply being immersed reduces *edema*, or swelling. That's a good enough reason to head to the pool right now. Being in the water returns all that extra fluid in your feet, ankles, calves, and hands to your bloodstream, increasing the blood flow to your fetus. The deeper you are immersed, the greater the benefit. If you jog in water up to your chest, you'll have less swelling all over than if you jog in knee-deep water.

As soon as that fluid moves, you'll notice that you have the sudden urge to urinate. This is a good sign. It means that your fetus and kidneys are seeing more blood flow. So swimming reduces swelling, is easy on your heart, and is especially good for your fetus.

The one drawback to swimming is that, since it is not a weight-bearing activity, it doesn't strengthen your bones and give you the labor and delivery benefits of, say, walking or hiking. The best pregnancy workout program combines a few swimming sessions per week with a few walks or jogs.

Even if you have never done much swimming before, there are lots of safe, shallow water activities you can enjoy, like water aerobics. You don't even have to go near the deep end. Plenty of community pools offer prenatal water activities and swimming courses—and you can continue some of these with your newborn. After all, your baby is a natural-born swimmer.

Especially if you have bad knees, are experiencing back pain, or have gained a lot of weight, water exercise is for you. If you have your own pool or have a chance to splash around in a lake or ocean, slather on the waterproof sunscreen and try jogging through waist-deep calm water. You can try many of the same activities you enjoy on land in the water, like jogging, walking, jumping, kickboxing, and even practicing your golf swing. The resistance of the water will give your muscles an excellent workout. And if that isn't enough, use some water weights to add resistance while you exercise in the pool.

Climbing into the water, you experience something like the peaceful aquatic environment your fetus is living in right now. The soothing, meditative rhythm of swimming also helps clear your mind. In many cultures, immersion also has special significance during pregnancy, symbolizing cleansing and regeneration.

RISK ASSESSMENT BY TRIMESTER

1ST TRIMESTER: LOW
2ND TRIMESTER: LOW
3RD TRIMESTER: LOW

swimming

Staying Healthy Each Trimester

1ST TRIMESTER | RISK: LOW

Even if you've never been much of a swimmer, you may decide to take up swimming or water aerobics this trimester for a number of reasons. First, you may not have the energy to do a whole lot else and swimming is an easy activity to take up, even if you're not very fit in the first place. Second, what better time to get into a swimsuit than when you're supposed to be gaining weight and getting round around the middle?

Third, establishing a swimming schedule early in pregnancy will really pay off down the road with greater confidence in the water and better physical condition. Women who take up swimming (or other non-weight-bearing exercise, like cycling) during early pregnancy are more likely to keep it up into their third trimesters.

If you begin to feel too warm or short of breath, slow down. Try floating on your back while catching your breath; this will build your abdominal and back muscles while giving your heart and lungs a rest. If nausea is keeping you out of the pool, eat a small, nutritious snack, like a banana, half an hour before swimming so that you have something in your stomach but are not too full.

When you're just starting out, try a fifteen-minute water workout, plus a five-minute warm-up and a five-minute cooldown. Mix up your workout so that you are doing some aerobics, some kicking, and some laps. If you are an experienced swimmer, include several strokes so that you are working all your muscles: the breaststroke works your arms, chest, and inner thighs; the freestyle or crawl stroke works your arms and buttocks; and the backstroke works your abdominals and upper back.

2ND TRIMESTER | RISK: LOW

If you swam during your first trimester, you'll still be comfortable in the water even with your growing belly, shifting center of gravity, and unusual buoyancy. Even if you have just decided to switch to swimming this trimester (from hiking, biking, or simply working too much), you'll adjust easily and get a good workout in the water. Plus, with your nausea out of the way and more energy this trimester, you can focus on exercising regularly and maintaining your stamina.

I never really exercised before I was pregnant, so I didn't think this was the time to start anything strenuous. My doctor recommended swimming, so I joined a prenatal swim class.

I would absolutely recommend swimming to other pregnant women. I've always loved water and I'm glad I started going to this class. It feels more like a support group than an intimidating exercise class. Also, getting out and meeting other people has helped me to get my mind off all the things I panic about going wrong. I experienced a miscarriage a few months prior before I started this class, and I just didn't want to do anything but sit on the couch and pray everything would be okay. My instructor teaches only prenatal classes, so if any of us has a particular pregnancy concern or problem, she is able to help.

Also, she isn't a "zen guru." She makes us work. She is preparing us for labor and to take care of a baby.

Hopefully, I will be in better shape (physically and mentally) to handle labor and motherhood.

I love my swim class, not only for the exercise but also because I have met other pregnant women going through the same thing at the same time. And that's made me feel more confident and able to enjoy this big belly!

—Jamie, St. Augustine, Florida

swimming

A regular water workout this trimester will reduce your back pain by both stretching and strengthening your back and belly muscles. You'll also be able to exercise without the joint pain that you might develop with running or even hiking this trimester. Doing both land and water activity is even better for you than doing just one or the other. I don't mean you need to become a pregnant triathlete, but go for variety every week.

If you've been swimming regularly for a couple of months, gradually ramp up your workout this trimester until you are swimming continuously for half an hour. This is a lot easier to do if you divide up your swim into sets: freestyle for six lengths, kicking for six, breaststroke for six, and backstroke for six, for example. Or try a medley, where each length is a different stroke. Don't forget to warm up and cool down. Depending on your speed and comfort in the water, aim to swim between twenty and forty lengths (in a twenty-five-meter pool) for a good workout.

3RD TRIMESTER | RISK: LOW

Maybe you haven't managed to do much exercise yet and your girlfriend has just talked you into trying prenatal water aerobics. That's great. It's not too late to start and swimming is your best choice. I promise you'll heave a sigh of relief when you step into the water and feel the weight lifted off your back. Even just a half hour in the water this late in pregnancy will help build your stamina, flexibility, and strength and put you in great shape for delivery.

Swimming is much less tiring and much easier on your joints than walking this trimester. Plus, you'll really appreciate the effect on your ankle swelling. If you're having trouble balancing—your big belly can throw off your balance a bit—try hanging on to a kickboard (a foam board that supports your upper body) until you get accustomed to the water. Playing in the surf (or in water with big waves) is not a good idea, since you can lose your balance and fall and may have trouble getting up quickly.

Even if you've been very active this pregnancy, you'll get out of breath surprisingly quickly. This is because you have less oxygen reserve later in pregnancy, the water puts pressure on your chest, and your big belly makes it difficult to take deep breaths. Don't worry—your fetus is getting enough blood and oxygen. You may also notice some Braxton Hicks contractions. These are normal just rest until they go away.

Try water aerobics or water jogging, which may feel easier than swimming laps with a big belly. Simply pushing through the water gives you a workout with good resistance. Swim laps if you can, but think about using a kickboard, hand paddles, fins, or even a life jacket to improve your stability, especially in the ocean. Aim to be in the water for thirty minutes at a time, including warm-up and cooldown. Then get in the shade and hydrate.

Warming Up

Always warm up, either by doing some walking in the water or long, easy strokes across the pool. If you are having difficulty swimming continuously, try swimming for thirty seconds, then resting for thirty. Warm up for five minutes to slowly raise your heart rate and activate your muscles. Do a few shoulder circles, supported squats, and arm stretches to make sure your swimming muscles are limber (see chapter 6). Any prenatal water aerobics or swim class will have a warm-up built in.

Swimming Technique for Pregnancy

You don't have to be an expert swimmer to reap the many benefits of water exercise during pregnancy. One of these benefits is that swimming, even if you are slow, awkward, and stick to the shallow end, will improve your posture on land. Because the water supports you, you have better posture in the water and your body learns how to stand straight. And even playing in the water tones your muscles. But there are a couple of things for you to keep in mind when swimming.

Freestyle (crawl stroke), breaststroke (with your head in or above the water), sidestroke, and backstroke are safe and healthy strokes during pregnancy. Each stroke works different muscle groups. If you feel at all dizzy or light-headed doing the backstroke, try swimming belly down instead. Stay away from the butterfly stroke, which can severely arch your back and over-stretch your abdominal muscles.

Breathe in a regular pattern that corresponds to your stroke. If you are a beginner, you'll have to breathe every stroke. If you are very fit, you can breathe every other stroke during breaststroke and even every third stroke during freestyle. Avoid holding your breath for sprints or diving to the bottom of the pool. If you usually do flip turns at the end of your laps, continue to do so until your belly gets too big for you to curl into a tucked position comfortably.

Cooling Down

Although you won't feel sweaty and hot after a good water workout, you'll still need to cool down. Just do a couple of leisurely laps, focusing on stretching your arms and legs with each stroke and slowing your breathing. Take about five minutes to cool down. If you head over to the shallow end afterward, you can do some arm, shoulder, and neck stretches before you get out of the pool. Then towel off and stretch your pelvic and leg muscles (see chapter 7).

Equipment Considerations

As your breasts and belly grow, your usual swimsuit may not give you the support, comfort, or coverage you are looking for. You want a suit you won't have to constantly adjust while working out; a one-piece suit with a built-in bra works best. Maternity suits will give your belly plenty of room to grow.

If you're going to be working out in chlorinated or salty water, wear goggles to protect your eyes. For long hair, try a swim cap to reduce your drag (it'll make your workout easier) and keep the hair out of your eyes. If you want to focus your workout on your arms and upper back, use a pull-buoy between your thighs to keep your legs afloat. If you want to focus on your legs, hold on to a kickboard while kicking.

If you're heading outdoors for a swim, make sure you slather on plenty of SPF-30 waterproof sunscreen (and reapply after toweling)—those UV rays will burn your delicate skin even worse in the water. Ideally, apply sunscreen half an hour before hitting the water to allow it to soak in and protect you in the water.

Preparing for Difficult Situations

As long as you are a confident swimmer, you can work out wherever there is water: at the beach, a friend's pool party, or the lake. If you're just getting started, stick to swimming under the expert gaze of your instructor. Stay out of water that is too warm (above 86˚F). Watch out for sunburn, big waves, cold water, underwater hazards, and currents. If you travel, be aware that in other countries some lakes and oceans may be polluted and pools may not be well chlorinated and so are not so safe for swimming. If you are concerned about water cleanliness, check the U.S. government's Centers for Disease Control (CDC) website.

Planning Pointers for Pregnancy

1 Join a prenatal class. Even if you're a strong swimmer, a prenatal water exercise class will give you a complete workout. It's also a great way to meet other pregnant women and get support. Plus, you can be confident your instructor will watch out for you and will encourage you to be there regularly.

2 Mix it up. Ideally, your weekly workout routine will also include a weight-bearing exercise like walking or jogging. If you mix it up (say, walking twice a week and swimming twice a week), you'll get the cardiovascular, strength, and flexibility benefits of both land and water exercise, while getting in the best possible shape for delivery. Plus, if you experience ankle swelling or joint pain after working out on land, swimming will help get rid of it.

3 Make it a habit. Swimming will tone your muscles, condition your heart and lungs, and keep you relaxed and positive—but only if you do it regularly. Keep it up after pregnancy too.

4 Love your body. Exercising is great for your growing fetus, but it's also good for your body and your self-esteem. Simply getting into a swimsuit and allowing the water to carry your weight will give you more confidence about your body and appreciation of the burden it is bearing. Invest in a cute maternity suit so you can show off the bulge!

swimming

5 Pick clean, cool water. Make sure the pool (or beach or lake) you swim in is clean. Any public pool in the United States should be well chlorinated (the chlorine won't hurt your fetus) to prevent infection. The water temperature should be between 82°F and 86°F (28°C and 30°C).

6 Beware of the sun. Being in or near the water outdoors almost guarantees you a sunburn if you're not very careful. Apply SPF-30 waterproof sunscreen and reapply every time you get in the water or towel off.

7 Splash around. Swimming is fun and very safe for you and your growing fetus. Run, crawl, kick, and float around. There is almost no better way to relieve the fatigue, swelling, and muscle aches of pregnancy than by spending some time in the water—and your baby will enjoy splashing around as much as you will.

snorkeling

If you are a reasonably good swimmer and are heading off to a beach destination, you might enjoy snorkeling as a way to explore the underwater world. Snorkeling is a safe and healthy combination of swimming and sightseeing. If you've done a bit of swimming during this pregnancy, you should have little trouble keeping your balance in the water and enjoying yourself. But if the idea of being far from shore or breathing through a pipe doesn't feel comfortable, take in the view from shore instead.

Like swimming, snorkeling offers the benefits of good aerobic exercise, a solid muscular workout, the relief of being off your feet and not carrying your own weight, and reduction of joint and muscular pain and swelling. Plus, you soar above the scenery but don't have to worry about falling or overheating.

But snorkeling does have its risks. Since you don't have the side of the pool to hold onto, you need to watch out for getting too far from shore or your boat. Turn back well before you start to feel tired or develop a cramp. Always snorkel with a buddy who is a strong swimmer and will look at for you or even hold hands while snorkeling. Wear a life jacket (or personal flotation device) so you don't get as worn out. Take frequent breaks out of the water to catch your breath, reapply sunscreen, and drink lots of water.

If you're swimming above coral, you won't be able to touch down, even in shallow water (touching coral will scratch you badly and will kill the coral). Make sure you will be able to get off and on the boat without jumping or diving. Before you take off, just check for a ladder off the side.

You may need to urinate more than usual as you snorkel—that's because immersion helps get rid of retained water and puts some gentle pressure on your bladder. But you still need to drink lots of water to replace the fluids lost due to direct exposure to the sun, exertion, and perspiration. Breathe slowly and regularly and don't hold your breath—even if you see a big fish. If you become anxious and short of breath, tread water, take off your mask and snorkel, look toward land, and get your bearings. And avoid free diving during pregnancy, even during your first trimester, because it may divert blood flow away from your uterus.

Unless you are lucky enough to live right near a great snorkeling site or are a marine biologist and snorkel for work, you will probably go snorkeling once or twice at most during pregnancy. That's okay, as long as you maintain a regular exercise regimen the rest of the time. The best exercise plan for pregnancy includes walking or running and a water activity, like swimming or water aerobics.

If you haven't exercised much this pregnancy, you'll be surprised to find how different your body feels in the water—your big belly really changes your buoyancy. And you'll notice that you get short of breath and tired more easily. Start by doing a little swimming in relatively shallow water. If you are still eager to do some snorkeling after that give it a try in waist-deep water with a sandy bottom first.

RISK ASSESSMENT BY TRIMESTER

1ST TRIMESTER: LOW
2ND TRIMESTER: LOW
3RD TRIMESTER: LOW

Staying Healthy Each Trimester

1ST TRIMESTER | RISK: LOW

Like swimming, snorkeling is a low-risk activity early in pregnancy. Although you may feel somewhat more out of breath and fatigued, your balance and buoyancy in the water aren't much different than before pregnancy. With a pair of fins and some good waterproof sunscreen, you'll be set to go.

If nausea bothers you when on the boat or while floating—you can get seasick just being jostled by surface waves—try eating a small snack (like a banana) half an hour before your excursion so that you are not hungry but not too full. When you're in the water, keep your eyes on the horizon and just tread water and look toward land for a few minutes to steady yourself. Drink water in smaller amounts, more often. Try snorkeling right around the boat so you can pause for a drink every ten minutes.

You need to stay cool in the water, so make sure the water temperature is between 82°F and 86°F (28°C and 30°C). A local dive shop will be able to tell you the exact water temperature. If the water is cooler than 82°F, wear a wetsuit. If the water is warmer than 86°F, as it may be in some tropical locations, stay out of it—it's too warm for your developing fetus.

With some serious sunscreen—or, better yet, a long-sleeved t-shirt—in place, you'll be able to stay out up to forty-five minutes at a time this trimester. Put your head up regularly to check your orientation and proximity to shore. It's okay if you are ready to head in to shore after just a few minutes if you are tired, uncomfortable, or just not feeling up to it. Take frequent breaks on deck for hydration and to give your body a rest without worrying about stepping on coral or a field of sea urchins.

2ND TRIMESTER | RISK: LOW

Snorkeling is really fun during your second trimester because your nausea has resolved and you've got the energy to get out there and see some fish. Simply being in the water will take a lot of strain off your back and you'll feel a lot better after snorkeling, especially if you have achy joints and muscles and swollen ankles. The gentle swimming—mainly light kicking—you do while snorkeling stretches and activates those tired muscles in your back and legs. Since you'll feel a little off balance because of your belly, always wear a life jacket and fins.

Taking regular breaks is especially important later in pregnancy. You can easily lose track of time because you feel so cool and relaxed while snorkeling, allowing you to become dangerously dehydrated and sunburned. Limit your snorkeling to twenty-minute excursions, interrupted by brief breaks for refueling if you're eager to hop back in.

3RD TRIMESTER | RISK: LOW

If you haven't tried swimming at all this pregnancy, your increased buoyancy will surprise you. Practice swimming in a shallow, sandy-bottomed area before putting on your snorkel gear. And put on some fins and a life vest, too. Then stick to chest-deep water with sandy patches where you will be able to stand to take a breather. Swimming or snorkeling in shallow water will also give you a good workout and give your back and legs a real break from carrying that heavy load—even if you don't see a lot of fish.

The snorkel may make you feel claustrophobic, even though you will be able to get enough air. Breathe slowly and regularly. This trimester, your growing belly puts pressure on your diaphragm, making it harder to get a deep breath in ordinary circumstances. This, combined with the water pressure, can make you feel like you're not breathing enough. Your fetus will get the oxygen it needs, but

"Snorkeling was the highlight of our last island vacation. Since I was seven months pregnant, diving was out of the question, but there was no way I was going to pass up the underwater scenery in Bonaire. Other than a few flamingoes on land, the real beauty of the little Dutch island is underwater in the marine park.

Although I'd done some swimming in the first few months of pregnancy, I hadn't been in the water recently. It was hilarious. My husband said I looked like a panicking five-year-old learning to dog-paddle. I felt awkward and I was splashing too much to see any fish.

Our guide thought a life vest and fins would help. And it did. With the extra buoyancy and power, I maneuvered around all right. For a while, I hung onto an inner tube, but I abandoned it once I got the hang of the water. I was worried that somehow the snorkel would restrict my breathing, but I didn't really notice a difference.

Floating effortlessly felt good. I felt like a soundless airplane gliding above the bustling coral cosmos. We saw turtles, cleaning stations, big-lipped groupers, and spectacular coral. Needless to say, I dragged my husband out snorkeling at least once a day.

—Leticia, Detroit, Michigan

if you feel uncomfortable, just take off the snorkel, put it around your neck or upper arm, and swim in to shore.

Keep an eye on the time you spend on the water, so that you are getting out of the sun regularly (at least every twenty minutes) to hydrate. Even with a life jacket and fins, you are getting a good workout and you're sweating off a lot of fluid. Listen to your body and don't let the fish tempt you too far from your boat or the shore.

Warming Up

Before heading out to see the fish, warm up on shore by doing a set of shoulder circles, supported squats, and arm stretches so that your swimming muscles are ready to go. Wading out from shore will also help warm up your legs. If you're snorkeling from a boat, the water will probably be deep enough for you to be able to slowly paddle around for five minutes, activate your arms and legs, and get used to the water. Just don't wear yourself out during the warm-up.

Snorkeling Technique for Pregnancy

Snorkeling is gentle exercise and slow, easy floating with a minimum of kicks is the best way to see marine life. While snorkeling you may feel like a sightseer, but you're also reaping the many benefits of water exercise. As you glide along, you keep your abdominal muscles firm, your kicking works your buttocks and thighs, and your back anchors your neck and arms. Your posture in the water is comfortable for you, since it takes the weight of your belly off your legs, and healthy for the pregnancy, since gravity pulls the uterus off of the major blood vessels that feed the fetus. The muscles you use to stay afloat (even with a life vest on) help your posture on land, too.

Once you get the hang of floating—with the help of fins, a life vest, and perhaps even a floating mat—take a few minutes near shore or near the boat to get a feel for breathing through the snorkel. If you are an experienced snorkeler, you are used to hearing yourself breathe and clearing your snorkel with a forceful blow to remove water. If this is your first time snorkeling, it may take a few minutes of standing, adjusting the mask, and experimenting with holding your face underwater before you're comfortable. The claustrophobia will pass as soon as you become entranced by the scenery. Avoid diving down to look under coral shelves or pick up starfish: holding your breath is harder and more dangerous during pregnancy because your respiratory rate is higher and it may temporarily reduce your fetus's oxygen levels; plus, most marine life is more active when undisturbed.

Cooling Down

Before crashing on the towel and swapping tales of fish sightings, take five minutes to cool down. Tread water near the boat or swim in to shore with some slow, easy strokes. Focus on stretching your arms and legs with each stroke and slowing your breathing. Once on deck or dry land, towel off and do some arm, shoulder, pelvic, and leg stretches before replenishing your fluids.

Equipment Considerations

I highly recommend wearing a life jacket, or personal flotation device, while snorkeling. Even strong nonpregnant swimmers wear them when snorkeling for several reasons. One, the bright color of a life jacket is easy to spot from far away, even in choppy water, so that boat personnel and your partner can keep an eye on you. Two, the life jacket will allow you to take frequent floating breaks so you won't get too worn out from swimming and treading water. Three, the vest will protect you from getting a nasty sunburn on your back. Four, the better your skin is covered, the better you are protected against painful scratches from coral, stings from floating jellies, and nips from curious fish. (A light bodysuit will protect against stings and sunburn in warm water and, in cooler water, a wetsuit will give you lots of added buoyancy and make swimming easier.)

Underneath, wear a swimsuit that supports your growing breasts and belly both in the water and out. Try a one-piece with a built-in bra and extra room for your belly. Make sure you have a good pair of fins. With your feet swelling and the ligaments in your feet relaxing, your old pair or usual size may feel too tight. Try a size bigger.

Get an easy-to-read waterproof watch to help you keep track of time so that you limit your snorkeling and sun exposure and take regular breaks. Your old snorkel and mask, or ones you rent at a local shop, will work just fine. Don't skimp on the sunscreen. Your skin, even more delicate during pregnancy, will punish you later if you don't protect it well—and often—on the water. I'm talking about waterproof SPF-30 sunscreen that you reapply early and often—every time you step out of the water. And wear a t-shirt or life vest to save your back from blisters.

Preparing for Difficult Situations

Use your best judgment before heading out on the water. Big waves, swells, currents, an impending storm, lightning, and water hazards, like fire coral or stinging jellies, are obvious risks. If you can, go with a guide who will help you visit the best sites, look out for dangers, and offer expertise. Remember, the ocean is not an aquarium. Don't touch the fish, plants, and coral—reactions to stings may be more pronounced during pregnancy, though not more dangerous. Make sure you are a confident swimmer and are comfortable with your equipment. If you have misgivings, stay on deck and enjoy the lovely scenery from above. Or try a floating mat with a window that allows you to see underwater.

Planning Pointers for Pregnancy

1 Plan ahead. If you are lucky enough to be heading to a tropical destination where you might snorkel, join a prenatal swim class several months ahead of time. This way, you'll be very comfortable in the water and confident about your body when you get there.

2 Stick with a group. Snorkeling with a guide is very educational. It doesn't mean you have to go where the crowds are, but it does mean that you'll see some interesting fish that you might otherwise miss (like a hiding eel or octopus) and have an experienced person nearby at all times. Also, choose a responsible partner who will watch out for you and remind you to take breaks and hydrate often.

3 Practice first. If you haven't been swimming or snorkeling yet this pregnancy, make sure you test your comfort level in the water and with the equipment before heading out on a boat. Swim around in waist-deep water with a sandy bottom so you can stop, stand, and adjust. Your buoyancy and stamina are very different than they were a few months ago and it'll take some practice for you to become comfortable.

4 Gear up with fins and a flotation vest. If you're wearing this gear, you'll swim faster, tire less quickly, and see more fish (if you're not splashing around trying to stay afloat, the fish won't be scared off). Plus, you'll be protected from sunburn on your back and you'll be more visible from shore.

5   No free diving. It is simply not a good idea to hold your breath during pregnancy, since you want to maintain a constant, healthy oxygen supply to your fetus. Resist the temptation to free dive, and avoid the extra exertion of sprinting or snorkeling without fins.

6   Stay away from challenging swims. Swimming against currents and big swells and going on long-distance snorkels (like around a bay), really tax your muscles and don't give you a chance to take breaks and recover. Stick with snorkeling in a calm area around the boat or near shore.

7   Heads up. Periodically look up to orient yourself to the shore, the waves, and the boat. It's easy to lose track of where you are when you're following fish.

8   Relax. You'll have a much more enjoyable snorkel and won't get worn out as quickly if you take it easy and let those big fins do most of the work. Breathe slowly and regularly. If you feel short of breath or freaked out, tread water, take off the snorkel, and reorient before putting your head back under or heading back to the boat.

9   Take breaks. Use the side of the boat, sandy patches, or your flotation vest to support you while you catch your breath and hydrate—at least once every twenty minutes.

snorkeling

10 Maintain a comfortable temperature. Since water conducts heat off your body very rapidly, you can begin to feel cold and shivery even in warm water. Get out, towel off, drink some water, and warm up. Don't get too warm, though. Make sure the water temperature is between 82°F and 86°F (28°C and 30°C).

11 Protect yourself from the sun. Even though you can't feel it while you're snorkeling, your skin is absorbing those reflected UV rays and you can suffer badly if you're not well protected. Your skin is very susceptible to sunburn during pregnancy and snorkeling is a guaranteed way to get too much sun. Wear a vest and t-shirt and slather on plenty of waterproof SPF-30 sunscreen (especially on the backs of your legs, neck, and arms) every time you dry off.

12 Sightsee. Snorkeling is an incredible adventure and no two snorkeling trips (or even two snorkelers' experiences at the same site) will be the same. You get a glimpse of a colorful, intricate, bustling world—and a break from this one. As long as you are a confident swimmer, get out there and enjoy the view.

scuba diving

If you're an ardent diver, you probably plan your vacations around note-worthy dive sites and seek remote and untouched pieces of marine paradise before the tourists discover them. Diving is for true adventurers who thrive on the adrenaline generated by being eighty feet underwater, encountering a rare leatherback turtle (they are twelve feet across), spotting restless sharks at twi-light, or coaxing a moray eel out of its hiding place. Although a good dive can feel as peaceful as a quiet hour spent in a great cathedral, it is a risky sport, espe-cially during pregnancy.

One of the risks of scuba diving is developing decompression illness, or the "bends," when ascending to the surface. This is a significant danger during pregnancy, because the fetus is particularly susceptible to decompression illness.

Decompression illness is caused by nitrogen bubbles in the bloodstream. If a diver resurfaces too quickly, nitrogen in the body bubbles into the bloodstream. These bubbles act like blood clots and affect every part of the body as they block off small blood vessels, causing joint pain, numbness, tingling, weakness, headache, confusion, shortness of breath, itching, and difficulty speaking. In a pregnant woman, the nitrogen bubbles can travel to the fetus, blocking blood flow, and possibly causing birth defects or even a miscarriage or stillbirth.

Although scuba diving is safe for healthy nonpregnant women, it is not recommended during pregnancy because of the real risks to the fetus. Even care-ful planning of the dives using dive tables and conservative depths is risky. After all, accidents happen, and being sixty feet underwater doesn't give you any room for error. Furthermore, unlike high altitude, diving simply hasn't been studied in pregnancy, so we are not well aware of all the potential dangers for the preg-nant woman or the developing fetus.

Since diving is such a common sport among young people, you may realize that you scuba dived before you knew you were pregnant. You are still likely to have a healthy pregnancy—but you should not dive again while pregnant. Take a safer approach and try snorkeling instead.

RISK ASSESSMENT BY TRIMESTER

1ST TRIMESTER: HIGH

2ND TRIMESTER: HIGH

3RD TRIMESTER: HIGH

paddling

Anyone who has been paddling before will tell you it's great fun. And it's not just for river rats. Paddling is rapidly gaining in popularity; city slickers, families, and—you guessed it—pregnant women are joining in. Why? Paddling is a sure way to escape the throngs on shore, explore new territory, and have a valid excuse for a water fight. Pregnant women rave that they feel weightless, agile, and liberated on the water. It's no wonder: the water takes the weight of pregnancy off your tired legs and feet and allows your upper body to get some exercise. Plus, if you pick your river well, you can sit back and let the current do most of the work. Or you can choose a lake or bay with stunning scenery and wildlife and quietly float as close to the wildlife as you can—to watch that sea otter crushing a crab with his nimble flippers or to explore that veiled passageway among the mangroves.

What *is* paddling, exactly? Paddling is characterized by sitting in a raft, kayak, or canoe and propelling oneself with a paddle. It sounds simple, doesn't it? Well, that's where the choices begin: what type of vessel to choose; what sort of water to attempt—river, sea, or surf; and where, oh where, to go. You can see paddlers everywhere, from Manhattan to the Amazon to Antarctica, from backyard streams to park ponds. The thing is, there are so many ways to enjoy paddling, so much variety, that you'll never have the same excursion twice.

Paddling enthusiasts are constantly pushing the limits of the sport, so common paddling activities—river kayaking, white-water rafting, and flat-water canoeing—have expanded to include sea kayaking, open-canoe surfing, and surf kayaking. (I won't even get into the extreme sports of kayaking waterfalls, river marathons, slalom, and kayak biathlons.) During pregnancy, your options are a little more straightforward, since you're looking to stay out of trouble. I recommend that you steer clear of ocean surf and Class-III (swift current with minor obstacles and substantial rapids which cannot be attempted without an experienced guide) or above rivers—even early in pregnancy. In both these conditions, the treacherous water can throw you overboard, flip you over, or scrape you along the bottom. Even a perfect Eskimo roll, executed as the result of years of training and practice, isn't healthy for your growing fetus. Think about it: you'll need to hold your breath, lean hard into your belly against the front of the kayak, and jerk your hips and back upright. Nope, it's just not a good idea during pregnancy.

But if you stick to gentle currents and calm shores, paddling is one of the safest and healthiest activities you can enjoy during pregnancy. Take your time and let the journey be your purpose. There is nothing as soothing as the rhythm of water lapping the side of your boat. Even late in pregnancy, you'll be able to paddle with ease and won't have to worry about falling or being jolted, as you would in other wilderness activities. Paddling is good exercise, too—it conditions your heart and lungs, builds stamina, and strengthens the muscles you use every day. As a result, you'll have extra energy and fewer aches and pains, and will feel better overall. And it's easy; you can learn the sport during pregnancy—even when your belly is big—and you can paddle at your own pace and even rest on the water, all while giving your tired knees and ankles a break.

If you are one of those few lucky women who live near a sound in the Northwest, a duck pond in the East, a wetland in the South, or a waterway just about anywhere and can get out to paddle several times a week, go for it! If getting to a meandering stream requires a weekend trip, you can include paddling as one activity among many. All kinds of other outdoor activities closer to home will get you in good shape for paddling, such as walking, swimming, and even biking. You can try a rowing machine to build your stamina. (Just keep in mind that, during your third trimester, pulling your elbows all the way back may become more difficult.) You really don't even have to be in great shape to paddle—it's gentle on your heart and muscles—and you'll enjoy yourself even on your first time out.

When planning a paddling excursion, just be sure that the conditions are safe so that you feel confident with your route. Even small changes in river flow (say, after rainfall or a dam adjustment) or tides can seriously affect your paddling conditions.

Climbing into your kayak, canoe, or raft, you'll experience an immense feeling of relief and relaxation. Imagine that this soft rocking is what your fetus feels inside her cocoon of amniotic fluid. The rhythm of paddling on the water as well as your awe-inspiring proximity to the wildlife—even in a pond in the middle of a city park, you'll find water birds and frogs—take your mind off other responsibilities and anxieties. This sense of peace, safe exercise, and time spent with friends and family are what you really need during pregnancy. And kayaking, rafting, and canoeing are activities your entire family can enjoy for years to come.

"

At the end of my first trimester, I needed a distraction from my rampant nausea and general feeling of being out of touch with the world. I was desperate. Pregnancy had not been what I had expected so far—I had spent much of it looking at the bottom of a bucket, hoping my retching would ease. Don't get me wrong—I was thrilled to be pregnant, but I just didn't feel like myself.

So when some old friends called me up to see if I was up for some river rafting, I knew this was my chance to get back in touch with my friends—and with myself. A daylong trip down the Snake River proved just the ticket. Planning the trip was half the fun and, as a result of our enthusiasm, appetites, and luck, we ended up with twice the food we could possibly eat and a perfect blue-sky day. We filled up the raft with ice chests of goodies (to my surprise—I have been a vegetarian for years—I developed a major craving for the fried chicken we had packed) and put in about twenty miles upriver.

Dragging my feet in the cold water of the river, feeling the gentle undulations of the raft, soaking up some sunshine, and gazing at bald eagles and snow-capped peaks returned a sense of peace I hadn't realized I was missing. My first trimester wore me out and all the outdoor activities I had previously enjoyed seemed impossibly beyond my sagging energy level. Rafting changed my perspective. All I did was float along and paddle a bit, but that river trip restored my sense of well-being and put me back in touch with a world I had been missing all those weeks curled up on the sofa.

—Jennifer, Jackson, Wyoming

"

RISK ASSESSMENT BY TRIMESTER

> **1ST TRIMESTER: LOW**
> **2ND TRIMESTER: LOW**
> **3RD TRIMESTER: LOW**

Staying Healthy Each Trimester

1ST TRIMESTER | RISK: LOW

Even if you haven't been very active before pregnancy, paddling is a great weekend activity to get you outdoors and motivate you to get in shape. It's easy on your heart and lungs, so you won't have that short-of-breath exhausted feeling you may experience early in pregnancy with land activities, like jogging. At first, you will need to think consciously about how to paddle and steer. But, the more often you paddle, the sooner you'll be able to forget about the mechanics and focus on the natural world around you.

Your morning sickness may interfere with plans to head out on the water, however. Some women feel queasy with the uneven rocking motion of the boat, especially early in the morning. If you find this is true for you, try eating a nutritious snack about half an hour before hitting the water or try sucking on a ginger candy when the nausea strikes. Staring at the bow of your boat, especially if you are tired, may make you feel ill. If motion sickness bothers you, remember to keep paddling—sitting still on rolling waves can make you queasy—and look around you and at the horizon ahead of you.

One benefit of being in a boat is that the breeze over the water keeps you cool; splashing around in the water helps, too. Because getting too hot may affect your growing fetus, protect yourself from the sun, hop in the water to cool off when you get a chance, and choose a shady inlet or a dawn or dusk paddle instead of open water or mid-afternoon exposure.

If you are a beginner, head out with a group and, ideally, an expert guide, on flat water. A one-day lesson will teach you invaluable safety tips and basic technique. Take time to warm up, take breaks, drink water (one liter for every hour of exercise), and cool down while out on the water so that you don't get worn out too quickly. Initially, paddle for half an hour at a time; this means handing off your paddle or stopping every half hour for a genuine break.

paddling

If you are an experienced paddler, stick with conditions well below your usual level—seek peace of mind rather than thrills. This trimester, as your stamina improves, you may be able to handle paddling for up to two hours at a time, hydrating and resting along the way.

Taking up paddling or other non-weight-bearing activities like swimming early in pregnancy means that you are much more likely to stay active and be in better shape well into your third trimesters.

2ND TRIMESTER | RISK: LOW

You may find that paddling is easier and more fun this trimester because you don't have to worry about nausea. Plus, your body is more accustomed to the pregnancy, so you may really have the energy to get out there and do some exploring.

As your fetus grows, you'll notice that your shifting center of gravity affects your balance in the boat. For this reason, a wider and longer boat may feel safer than the zippy, maneuverable smaller boats. By the middle of the second trimester, many women prefer double kayaks over singles, for several reasons. First, the wider cockpit makes getting in and out of the kayak easier. Second, the double feels much more stable on the water than a single does. Third, riding in a double means you have your partner's help keeping up with the rest of the group and can take breaks without falling behind.

Because your joints are somewhat relaxed during pregnancy, some joint injuries are more common. The best protection is to warm up before heading out and to stretch on the water when your back and shoulders feel tired. If you have wrist problems—carpal tunnel syndrome is more common during pregnancy—wrist splints may help. If your lower back and legs begin to complain, head to shore and get out of the boat to give your lower body a stretch, too.

Unless you are extremely fit, limit your paddling sessions to an hour at a time (hydrating along the way, as always). Breaking after an hour will give you a chance to stretch, relax your arms, drink water, and get something good to eat. Any paddling trip during pregnancy should include real breaks—not just flat water—and a conservative distance plan. You may float fifteen miles downriver on a big raft in an afternoon but be completely worn out paddling one mile in a choppy estuary; have an alternative plan handy and stick close to shore so you can take unplanned rest stops.

3RD TRIMESTER | RISK: LOW

Flat-water canoeing, kayaking, and rafting are still very safe activities during your third trimester.

If you've been paddling before, you'll notice a few changes this trimester as your belly really grows. For one, you have less upper-body mobility, meaning it's harder to turn your torso to the side with each forward stroke. Therefore, your arms do more work—and get tired more easily. Many women in the third trimester prefer shorter paddles that require less rotation. Sitting for long periods may also become uncomfortable—your tailbone can be quite tender by your third trimester. You may want to stick closer to shore, where you can get out of the boat to stretch periodically.

Your bladder is also squeezed underneath that big belly, so you'll need to urinate more often than you'd like. Do not, I repeat, do not dehydrate yourself to avoid peeing. When you're on the water, sweating and exercising in the sun, you need more fluids than ever. And, dehydration is dangerous during pregnancy, especially this trimester, when it can stimulate contractions. But you can try several clever solutions to the urination problem. You can just hop onshore when you have to go. You can hop in the water (even in your wetsuit) and let the cool water stimulate your bladder. Or you can carry a "handheld urinary director" (a small cup with a tube attached to a bag) which allows you to pee while seated in the cockpit. To make this easier, try a man's wetsuit with zippers in the right places or make sure your clothes have the access you need.

This trimester, you'll need to take more frequent breaks to relieve cramped muscles and empty your bladder. Paddle for half an hour at a time, with brief breaks out of the boat to stretch your legs and back. Keep some healthy snacks handy and drink at least a liter of water for every hour you are outdoors.

Warming Up

Before you get comfortable in your boat, warm up the muscles you are going to use and stretch so you don't become cramped after the first fifteen minutes. Walking on shore for ten minutes will get your heart pumping, especially if you are helping to carry gear to the water (protect your back when lifting). Try some dynamic stretches to activate your arms, back, and hips (see chapter 6). "Windmilling" or "air paddling" will also warm up your arms and shoulders.

paddling

Once you're balanced in your boat and have your gear stowed, you can do some more stretches—especially if you start to feel cramped on the water. Stretch your hamstrings by leaning forward toward the bow of the boat. Hold for twenty seconds, and release. Paddling really works your upper body, so stretching your torso is important; holding your paddle in your hands in front of you, parallel to the water, turn to the side so your entire upper body is facing the side of the boat. Then turn the other way. Repeat three times on each side. If your wrists feel tired, put down your paddle and use one hand to pull back the fingers toward your forearm so the wrist is fully extended. Repeat on the other side. Then start paddling with slow, easy strokes to establish your rhythm on the water.

Paddling Technique for Pregnancy

Every boat and paddle require slightly different technique. When you're a beginner, the subtle differences don't matter much, since you're still mastering how to use your body efficiently. Even so, you're in great shape to paddle during pregnancy. Why? You don't need brute force to move quickly. The more relaxed you are, the more flexible your body will be and the less likely you'll be to cramp up and poop out. Quick bursts of energetic paddling—to chase a fleeing egret, for example—will just wear you out and aren't the best way to see wildlife anyway. Instead, practice a regular stroke that you'll be able to keep up for an hour or so.

You'll also find that your lower center of gravity during pregnancy improves your balance and stability. If you feel tippy with your jerky strokes, a steady paddling rhythm will also help keep your boat flat on the water and give you rock-solid balance. Plus, pregnancy gives you additional agility in your hips, which is helpful for steering and controlling the boat under you.

Pregnancy is a great time to focus on your form, especially if you have some bad paddling habits to break. For example, if you just use your arms to paddle, you'll become worn out pretty quickly. Instead, use your whole body to power your strokes. A little instruction can help you develop an efficient stroke.

Balance is a function of posture. Sit up straight in your boat and point your belly button out toward the front of the boat, so that your neck and buttocks are aligned. This posture helps your pelvis roll forward slightly so that it is anchored to your seat, it braces your thighs against the deck, and it pulls up your vertebrae so they are resting one on top of the other. Sitting up straight improves your range of motion dramatically. You'll be able to turn your entire torso from side to side, keeping your arms in front of you. Your forward stroke should then be close to the side of the boat and come out of the water next to your hip. This way, you rely on your torso muscles, reducing back and shoulder strain and boosting your power with each stroke. If you hit a rough patch, lean forward to improve your stability. Leaning back or slouching will throw you off balance, strain your back, and result in an inefficient stroke.

Take care to maintain good technique during pregnancy because your joints are more vulnerable to sprains. During paddling, keep an eye on your wrists. Hold your wrists straight so that they don't bend from side to side or back and forth. In a canoe, sit comfortably with your knees below the gunwales (the edges of the boat) so that you don't have to lift your paddle over your knee with each stroke. Sitting is far more comfortable than kneeling. However, if you hit rough water and have to get lower in the boat, kneel with your knees pushed as far out to the sides as is comfortable; consider using a pad to kneel on and a pillow between your thighs and lower legs to help support your weight.

In a kayak, make sure you have good back support and plenty of room for your legs so that your feet are on the footrests and your knees open out into a diamond shape. If your legs aren't comfortable, you can strain your hips when turning and end up pretty sore by the end of the morning. A relaxed position gives you extra stability and allows you to use your knees to maneuver the boat (lifting a knee rocks the kayak in the opposite direction).

One of the hardest things about paddling can be transporting your boat, especially during pregnancy, when you have to be extra careful not to strain your back. The easiest solution is to travel with a partner or group or rent near your put-in location. A boat cart is also useful. I do not recommend portaging (carrying your boat from one waterway to another); it's just too strenuous.

Cooling Down

If the weather and water are comfortably calm and warm, you can go for a refreshing dip at the take-out site. Ten minutes of easy swimming in the water will really stretch out those tired arm and shoulder muscles. Plus, a little dip will help get the blood flowing to your legs and help reduce any ankle and foot swelling from sitting still for a couple of hours. Then try a few stretches, focusing on your shoulders, arms, back, and pelvis, to prevent soreness and keep you limber for your next paddling excursion.

paddling

Equipment Considerations

Once you've spent some time on the water, you'll get a sense of what equipment is just right for you. (But remember, the type of equipment is never as important as good posture and good planning.) During pregnancy, you may want to make a few minor adjustments to the equipment you have.

Padding the cockpit is a way for you to support the joints and muscles that can bother you during pregnancy. For example, padding the seat so that it is flatter—not slanted backward—can reduce back strain. In a kayak, the built-in thigh braces may also become uncomfortable as your weight increases—you may need less "hook" in the brace. Beginner kayaks tend to have less hook and may feel more comfortable. As your belly grows, you can use pre-cut hip pads (you can get these at a kayak outfitter or cut a wedge-shaped canoe knee pad in half) to improve your fit. The more snugly you fit, the easier it will be for you to control your turns.

You'll be safest on your own, familiar boat. But if you're downgrading to flat-water paddling from surfing or white-water, you may have to turn in your craft for something that fares better on smooth, shallow water.

If you're going canoeing, you'll be in good shape in a short, wide boat. These are generally more maneuverable, though slower, than long, skinny canoes. Although a flat-bottomed boat may seem more stable initially, it is more likely to flip over if you hit turbulent water. Your best bet—except in perfectly calm, obstacle-free water, like a pond—is a rounded or V-bottomed hull, which is more predictable and resists capsizing. Having a keel or a V-bottom will also help the boat run straighter. Good boat choices for pregnancy are expedition (touring or tripper) canoes, which are very stable, and recreational canoes, which are designed for flat water and are easier to turn.

If you'll be kayaking while pregnant, try a touring kayak. Touring kayaks, longer than regular river kayaks, are sleek, fast, stable, and easy to paddle. Unlike canoes, they sit low in the water and have a covered deck, so you feel steadier in choppy water, are less affected by crosswinds, and stay drier. Plus, the cockpits are roomier, which means you don't have to worry about getting stuck if the kayak flips. In general, the wider the profile of the boat on the water, the more stable and reliable it will feel.

If you're a beginner or weekend paddler, you don't have to worry much about the incredible variety of paddles out there—just go with what the rental offers you. Don't even think about cupped and flat power faces, the taper on the fine-edging of a paddle, straight versus S-shaped blades, offset palm grips, or shaft flex until you're an undeniable paddle freak and you're ready to talk business. Until then, the only technical detail you need to worry about is size: a smaller paddle blade provides more fluid shock absorption and thus is easier on your arm muscles and joints.

There are a few other necessary pieces of equipment for paddling, and a life jacket, or personal flotation device (PFD), is certainly one of them. During pregnancy, you are more vulnerable to drowning because your lung capacity is less and your need for oxygen is greater. This makes a reliable, well-fitted PFD a must, even when you're just fooling around in shallow water. If it's cold, a wetsuit provides excellent protection. Finally, the more you cover up on the water, the better. The UV reflection on the water can really burn your skin and eyes if you don't wear a hat, sunglasses, and plenty of SPF-30 waterproof sunscreen.

Preparing for Difficult Situations

The best preparation for difficult situations is to plan to avoid them altogether. Rough water, strong winds, and unpleasant weather can ruin a fun day in the wilderness and put you at risk for heat exhaustion, cold exposure, overexertion, dehydration, injury, and worse. Make realistic adjustments to your paddling plans during pregnancy; plan for breaks and a shorter trip. Choose straightforward, flat-water conditions, even in early pregnancy and even if you are an expert. No curdling white water and no foaming surf. Check the currents and tides so that your return trip is down current. Talk with local rental shops to find out the most current conditions and the classification of the river (remember, you should be in rivers designated Class II—slowly flowing water with some waves and minor rapids which require little maneuvering—and below during pregnancy).

Overnight trips into the wilderness are possible during your first trimester if you are an experienced paddler and camper (see chapter 9 for tips on camping while you're expecting). Just avoid destinations that require carrying your boat and gear over land.

If you are heading down a rocky river, even if the water is relatively calm, wear a helmet in case you get thrown overboard (from a raft) or flip over (in a canoe or kayak). Be aware that some lakes and shore areas are polluted, so may not be safe for swimming. If you are concerned about water cleanliness, check with the U.S. government's Centers for Disease Control (CDC) website.

Planning Pointers for Pregnancy

1 Take a class. A couple of hours of professional instruction or a basic paddling course will give you confidence on the water, teach you the basics of good form and water safety, and be fun any time during pregnancy.

2 Paddle for health. Paddling is an excellent aerobic exercise that is also gentle on your joints. It's a great way to get fit during pregnancy and improve your stamina, flexibility, and cardiovascular health. Plus, it's one of the few sports that allows you to forget about your bulky pregnant body and dance across the water gracefully. The best way to get in shape for paddling (and for delivery) is by doing it often—throwing in some weight-bearing exercise like walking or hiking to round out your routine.

3 Know how to get help. While paddling, you'll be drawn to stray far from crowds, park headquarters, and medical facilities—getting away from it all is the whole point. However, especially during your third trimester, make sure you are able to get help if you need it. Routes along shore and river passages that run parallel to a road are safest. Some parks have cell phone service. Always let someone at your put-in site know where you are headed and when you will be returning.

4 Pick a stable craft. Whether you decide to raft, kayak, or canoe, make sure you feel confident in your boat. The better your boat fits you, the easier navigation will be. In general, a short, wide boat is more reliable than a long, narrow one. As your belly grows, you may find that shorter, smaller paddles are easier to use as well.

5 Go double. A double kayak, canoe, or raft allows you to have more stability, support, and sheer power if you need it. You also enjoy the companionship of your partner or a friend with whom you can share the adventure. Plus, you may need that help getting the boat in and out of the water in the first place.

6 Always wear a PFD. A good life jacket is meant to save your life, but it also serves several other useful functions: it keeps the sun off your back, it can make you more visible, and it allows you to go for a dip and float along in deeper water (with your feet out in front of you). The color is important. Green and brown will help you blend in when watching wildlife. Red and yellow are highly visible and perfect for high-traffic areas, such as around larger boats.

7 Choose cruising conditions. You want to be able to sit back and relax on the water. Let the warble of an exotic bird—rather than the roar of white water—get your adrenaline pumping. Stay away from waves, strong currents, and rivers designated Class III (substantial rapids requiring an experienced guide) and above during pregnancy.

paddling

8   Hydrate and urinate often. Yes, it is annoying to have to hop out of the boat frequently to pee, but staying hydrated is essential for your health and your fetus's health. Plus, you'll feel lousy and can get overheated if you don't drink enough.

9   Slow and steady wins the race. A natural paddling rhythm is easier on your heart, lungs, and muscles and will allow you to keep at it longer. Bursts of enthusiastic paddling will wear you out and scare away the birds.

10   Protect yourself from the sun. The steady sun from above and its reflected rays on the water can give you a terrible burn—especially during pregnancy when your skin is more vulnerable. Don't push off without wearing a wide-brimmed hat, sunglasses, and waterproof SPF-30 sunscreen.

11   Enjoy your paddle. Plan to see wildlife. Insist on relaxing. Paddling during pregnancy will give you a sense of freedom, speed, and weightlessness that is simply exhilarating. Although your first strokes in a boat may feel heart-stoppingly tipsy, I promise you'll get the hang of paddling and will be a graceful glider by the end of your first excursion. And it's a skill you'll use after you become a parent, since paddling is a real blast for kids, too.

boating

Whether they are partial to a yacht, a rowboat, a sloop, a catamaran, an outrigger, or a cabin cruiser, boaters are passionate about their sport and hesitate to give up boating, even during pregnancy. And there is little reason to. If you feel comfortable on your boat, the relaxation, fresh air, and company are good for you. While we can't pretend it's great exercise, lounging on deck and even helping with rigging does offer several bonuses: the thrill of sport; the fun of participating in a special event; and, often, the extra rewards of exploring, snorkeling, bird watching, fishing, and swimming.

Boating is a great way of getting outdoors during pregnancy, since you can spend a sporting afternoon with friends and family without worrying about getting short of breath or falling behind. Plus, most boats have radio contact so you can get help and be located at any time if you need it. Stay away from rough water, extreme temperatures, jet skis, racing, and risky wind conditions. Think mellow. Think flat water. There's not a whole lot else to it—except maybe packing a scrumptious picnic.

If you want to do something really healthy for your pregnancy, hop in! Getting in the water to splash around and cool off is especially good for your developing fetus. Swimming—or even dog-paddling with a life jacket on— conditions your heart and lungs and is an important part of getting fit for the rest of pregnancy, delivery, and parenthood. Round out your outings with some aerobic exercise too, like hiking or swimming, so your fetus can benefit as much as you do.

Boaters are undeniable outdoor enthusiasts and, often, the boat is just a means to an end: to get to the perfect secluded camping spot, the best bay from which to watch the sunset, the rock where the big fish gather, or the remote snorkeling reef. Or it might just provide a way to hang out in the middle of the lake, where you can tease the other boaters with the aroma of your barbecue.

RISK ASSESSMENT BY TRIMESTER

1ST TRIMESTER: LOW
2ND TRIMESTER: LOW
3RD TRIMESTER: LOW

boating

Staying Healthy Each Trimester

1ST TRIMESTER | RISK: LOW

During your first couple of months of pregnancy, morning sickness may rear its ugly head when you're snugly settled on the boat. Being inside the cabin, reading, talking, and focusing on parts of the boat, rather than the world around you, can make nausea worse. The solution is to get out on deck for fresh air and look toward the horizon—and land—to steady yourself.

Stay on the water as long as you are comfortable, but beware of the sun's effects on your delicate skin during pregnancy. Wearing cool cotton clothing and a big hat is a must on exposed decks at sea or in the middle of a lake or river. Wind and sun dry your sweat quickly, so you may not realize how much fluid you are losing and need to replenish. Keep an eye on the clock and monitor your hydration so that you are drinking sufficient amounts and need to urinate at least every four hours.

2ND TRIMESTER | RISK: LOW

Your growing pregnancy and shifted center of gravity this trimester may throw you off balance as the boat rides the waves. Hold onto handrails, wear shoes with good traction, and always wear a life jacket, or personal flotation device (PFD). Wearing a life jacket is imperative for several reasons: during pregnancy, you are more likely to lose your balance. If you land in the water, the shock of falling and the buoyancy of your belly can make it more difficult for you to orient yourself; you are also at greater risk for drowning with your decreased lung capacity and increased need for oxygen.

This trimester, with your energy up and your pregnancy in full swing, take advantage of being on the water to do something active. Take along snorkeling equipment or a dinghy so you can go exploring onshore. Limit your excursions to half an hour so you can replenish your fluids and calories regularly. If you're simply hanging out on deck, get into the shade or in the water at least once every hour to cool off.

3RD TRIMESTER | RISK: LOW

Keeping your balance is your primary challenge on the boat this trimester. Staying in calm waters if possible, anchoring yourself when walking, and wearing slip-proof shoes are key when moving around on slick, turbulent decks. Even if you're not tossed overboard, lurching forward and jamming your belly against a cooler is no good for the pregnancy.

Use the boat's ladder to get in and out of the boat; jumping and diving are not a good idea, even early in pregnancy, because of the direct impact to your belly and the risk of water forcefully entering your vagina.

At this point in pregnancy, you've probably experienced swelling around your ankles, and even around your legs and hands in warm weather. When sitting on deck, try to elevate your feet to relieve swelling. But, if you can, get in the water. Immersing yourself helps your body return that extra fluid back to your bloodstream—improving your circulation and getting rid of the swelling. It's also a perfect excuse to start a civil water fight.

Hydrate aggressively this trimester and limit your sun exposure to an hour at a time so that you don't become too sunburned or dehydrated. Keep in mind that you are also susceptible to both sunburn and dehydration and that wind can dry you out even on cloudy days.

Warming Up

If you're only using the boat to get from point A to point B or to enjoy an afternoon chilling on deck, you don't need to warm up. If your boating excursion develops into an adventure involving paddling, swimming, hiking, or other activities, you should take care to stretch and plan appropriately (take a look at the appropriate chapters for specific tips).

Boating Technique for Pregnancy

If you're on a small boat, you have the delicious sensation of being suspended right above the water, temporarily liberated from carrying your pregnancy weight but endowed with grace and speed. On a larger boat, you have the security of an enclosed deck, comfortable chairs, and shade. Even if you are not doing anything particularly active, you may want to check out some of the dynamic stretching (see chapter 6) and cooldown activities that you can practice on deck (on still water,

Summer arrived just as my belly was beginning to become visible (at least to me!) and my energy was coming back. I started to get really excited about my family's yearly trip to my grandparents' cabin on the lake. I was ready to share the news of my first pregnancy with the entire family and I knew I'd be treated like a queen.

I had a few doubts, though. I knew I wasn't up for the usual water skiing, but I wasn't too enthusiastic about slow baking in the sun on shore, either. I realized the perfect solution: hanging out on the boat. It was social, relaxing, low energy—and hilarious, since I could take over driving while the rest of the crew tried outrageous shenanigans on the water skis and the banana.

When we boated to the far shore for some fishing, I was happy to go along. I brought along a sun umbrella, a cushion, and a thermos of limeade. With my fishing pole suspended from the deck in front of me, I even caught a bass (although the smell of fish turned my stomach). With the gentle rocking of the boat and whirring of my brother's line, I also caught up on my sleep.

One evening, my mother and I took the boat out alone together to watch the sunset. In that peaceful time when the lake became golden, she told me about her own hopes and fears when she first became pregnant (she ultimately had five kids). Sharing that magical hour with my mother on the lake was very special to me because I was about to become a mama myself.

—Clarie, Portland, Maine

obviously). Stretching your back and legs several times an hour can relieve strain from sitting for long periods, especially in somewhat cramped quarters. Bring a cushion or two to sit on, to save your tailbone from hard deck chairs and seats.

If you're headed out for a longer journey, on a cruise ship or a live-aboard yacht, for example, frequent stretching is a great way to get your blood flowing, improve your posture and breathing, and even prevent blood clots and muscle aches. And you don't need a lot of space in which to do it.

Cooling Down

Cooling down and staying cool are key. If you're out boating on a warm day, whether you are exercising or not, make sure you stay cool with cold drinks, shade, and appropriate lightweight clothing.

Equipment Considerations

When you're boating, you may not have a lot of choice about the equipment, but you can bring along some useful accessories. A wide-brimmed hat, a lightweight cotton coverall or beach shirt, waterproof sandals or shoes with good traction, and several firm cushions will make you a lot more comfortable.

Wearing a life jacket, or personal flotation device, is a must. It also offers several advantages besides flotation, including high visibility on the water, the ability to reduce the direct impact to your belly if you fall, and good sun protection for your upper body. Just pick a bright color that agrees with you, and get a good fit.

Bring lots of water so you can stay well hydrated—the wind and sun will dry you out. Just pee over the side if you have to; it is unsafe to dehydrate yourself to avoid urinating while off shore. Dehydration can have serious consequences during pregnancy, including harming your fetus and stimulating labor contractions.

Your skin is particularly vulnerable to sunburn during pregnancy, so slather on the waterproof SPF-30 sunscreen and reapply every time you get wet—even with megasplashes—and every time you towel off.

Preparing for Difficult Situations

Any experienced captain will equip her boat with safety gear; if you are headed off shore, check for adequate life vests, a radio, and a flare *before* you push off. If you have any misgivings about the captain's abilities, the weather, or the boat, just get off. Rough waves, a drunken crew, an inexperienced skipper, unfamiliar waters, or ominous weather can ruin even a short boat ride.

Getting stranded on open water is a real risk and puts you, in particular, in danger of dehydration, overexertion, severe burns, heat illness, cold exposure, and worse. Know the distance you are going, the approximate time you'll be on the water, and the basic route. Find out whether other boats are headed the same way. Talk with local boaters or rental companies about the regional conditions and any anticipated changes, so you know what to expect, or whether to postpone the trip to another day.

Planning Pointers for Pregnancy

1   Know your captain. Make sure that you are confident of the skills and reliability of the crew and company that you are boating with. Familiarity with the waters, mindfulness of the weather, and attentiveness during the trip make a good captain.

2   Limit your exposure. Keep an eye on the time and the sun and get in the shade and in the water regularly; if you can, cool off every half hour. Protect yourself from wind, surf, and cold.

3   Wear a life jacket. During pregnancy, you are more susceptible to both falling in and drowning. The life jacket will keep you afloat if you fall into the water, and it also gives you good visibility from far away, a little insulation, and protection from the sun.

4   Hydrate regularly. Exposure to sun and wind dry you out fast. Drink at least a liter of water every hour and keep an eye on your urine to make sure it hasn't become dark with dehydration. With proper hydration you should need to urinate at least every four hours.

boating

6   Get active. Get wet. Take the opportunity of being on the water to swim, snorkel, paddle, or at least stretch and activate your sore muscles. Getting in the water provides a great workout, takes the strain off your back and legs, and helps relieve swelling.

Combat nausea. Being on the water, especially if you're not the one driving the boat, can worsen your nausea. Eat a nutritious snack, such as a banana, a half hour before getting on board. If nausea strikes while you're out, try sucking on a ginger candy and getting up on deck to watch the horizon.

7   Choose a gentle ride. Heading out on rough water is dangerous and will compound your nausea and unsteadiness. Instead, plan a relaxing outing on flat water where you can focus on the scenery rather than the strength of your grip on the rail.

8   Sunscreen. Constant exposure, the fierce reflection of the sun's rays off the water and the deck, and repeated splashing demand some tough waterproof SPF-30 sunscreen and frequent reapplications.

windsurfing

Windsurfing is an exhilarating combination of sailing and surfing.
It can be peaceful or downright spine-tingling. When the wind catches you, it will whisk you across an expanse of water before you can take a second breath. And if you're an experienced windsurfer, you'll know how to just hang on and enjoy the ride. It is delicious to experience that freedom from your heavy body during pregnancy—that moment of almost effortless flight.

If you are a strong windsurfer with years of wind wisdom and absolute confidence in your ability to handle your board, you can windsurf during early pregnancy. But don't strut your stuff. This is not the time for slashing a wave or getting air; even if you do them right, these moves are too dangerous during pregnancy. Aside from the obvious risk of injury, you may get drilled (held underwater) and have to hold your breath—and this just isn't healthy for your developing fetus.

Choose conditions at least several levels below your abilities. Why? The wind and water are powerful forces and you can easily become tangled with your equipment, pounded off the bottom in the sand, catapulted onto hard water, and caught off guard by a sudden gust—and end up underwater or injured. After your third month, when your uterus begins to grow up and out from behind the pubic bone, your fetus is even more vulnerable to injury, so I don't recommend windsurfing at all after the first trimester. Furthermore, your back bears the burden of the pregnancy and windsurfing can contribute to backaches. Finally, if you get stuck and need to lie facedown on your board and paddle in, your uterus is in the way.

Don't get me wrong: if you're experienced and skilled, I'm all for your enjoying some gentle windsurfing during your first trimester. And the swimming (or treading water) you do while getting your equipment in line or after wiping out is fantastic exercise also—and it really benefits your fetus. If you decide to windsurf, don't hesitate to hop in and swim a lot, too.

RISK ASSESSMENT BY TRIMESTER

1ST TRIMESTER: MEDIUM

2ND TRIMESTER: HIGH

3RD TRIMESTER: HIGH

windsurfing

Staying Healthy Each Trimester

1ST TRIMESTER | RISK: MEDIUM

I consider windsurfing to be a medium-risk activity during early pregnancy because it's only safe for experienced windsurfers. This is not a good time to learn to windsurf, even on placid water, because you are bound to take a lot of falls and the potential trauma (of equipment slamming on your belly or of water being forced inside your vagina) is not healthy for your pregnancy. If you're still taking the occasional catapulted dive or haven't gotten the hang of tacking windward and jibing, try practicing only on land during pregnancy. It's a great way to perfect basic skills and improve your form. Even basic maneuvers, such as uphauling, rotating the board, and controlling your movement in inconsistent conditions, require skill and sheer strength and pose risks to inexperienced windsurfers, especially pregnant ones.

Choose conditions conservatively and make sure the weather and water temperature are ideal. The water should be between 82°F and 86°F (28°C and 30°C). If the water is any warmer than that, then it's probably too hot outside also, and you can overheat more easily, which isn't good for your fetus. If it's chilly, you should consider wearing a wetsuit.

This trimester, you have to protect your fetus by not overexerting yourself—and by staying cool. This means taking breaks. I know this can be a challenge when you're on the water and the wind is consistent. If the conditions are good, the wind won't give you a break—but you still need to take one. Every fifteen minutes, hop off your board, cool off, and swim and stretch a little before getting going again.

If you're far from shore, float and hang onto your board for a break. And don't plan to windsurf for longer than an hour at a time; for most of us, just a half hour is a very good workout. After an hour or less, you need to come in to shore to hydrate, eat a snack, and reapply sunscreen to your sunburn-prone skin.

2ND TRIMESTER | RISK: HIGH

The unpredictability and power of the wind and water are what make windsurfing so challenging and addictive—and so dangerous. I don't recommend windsurfing after your first trimester, not only because of the risk of injury to your own rapidly changing body (just consider the added strain on your lower back) but because of the risk to your fetus as well. Your growing uterus can be injured in any falls, dives, and boom accidents you may have. Plus, you can't comfortably lie on your belly to paddle to safety if you needed to. Any one of these risks is a good enough reason for you to stay off the board and swim instead. Besides, swimming will better prepare you for the rest of your pregnancy and delivery anyway.

3RD TRIMESTER | RISK: HIGH

It would take a lot of confidence (and a potent windsurfing addiction) to tempt you on to your board this trimester. Windsurfing is just too dangerous this late in pregnancy—your fetus is just under the surface of that big belly. Even a purposeful jump into the water sends a harsh jolt to your uterus. You don't have to stay out of the water, though. Keep up your upper body strength and build your stamina by swimming or doing water aerobics in preparation for labor and delivery and a quick postpartum recovery.

Warming Up

Don't make your first fall your first dip into the water. Before you haul your board into the water, get in and swim for about five minutes to warm up your arms and to gauge the water temperature. Then get out and do some dynamic stretching to activate your arms and back (see chapter 6). Once you're warmed up, check your rigging and try to look graceful as you launch.

Windsurfing Technique for Pregnancy

Successful windsurfing is all about having a good stance. Not only will you look better sailing out there, but you'll also save your back—and you can't afford a back injury during pregnancy. You've probably heard this a hundred times before, but I'll tell you again: You need to keep your back straight. Bend your knees slightly and lean back a little to counterbalance the wind on the sail. This position will allow you to stay relaxed but remain alert to unexpected shifts in the wind. It also prevents awkward falls—like those where you take the mast down with you—and painful injuries.

"I've never been a really die-hard windsurfer, but this is Maui, and I hang out with plenty of work-all-night, windsurf-all-day types. I think the fact that I've always been pretty cautious allowed me to feel comfortable taking out my board—my fat ugly board—a few times during pregnancy.

The biggest hurdle, to be honest, was my own sheer laziness. I had gained weight and gotten out of shape, and I just didn't have much energy. But on a few occasions, while lying on the beach and trying to ignore the steady breeze, I had to throw in the towel and give it a go.

Getting tired easily kept me out of any big wind and my nausea kept me off the big waves. Although my previous windsurfing excursions lasted from what seemed like sun up to sun down, I was heading back to my towel after a mere half hour. Pathetic, but worth it.

Gone was my stamina. But it was replaced by a peaceful sense of balance on the board, like I was anchored from within. All I had to do was hang on and slip through the wind.

—Dawn, Maui, Hawaii"

Your arms, not your back, should do the work of sheeting in and out the sail. If you feel strain in your back while windsurfing, your stance is probably wrong; you may be leaning toward the sail or hunching your shoulders. The curved, sore back is the downfall of the beginning windsurfer. If you're not experienced, energetic, or fit enough to keep your back straight, head in to shore.

Keeping your balance is also key to windsurfing technique. If you are well balanced, you'll be able to handle turns and choppy water more easily. Plus, you'll be more hydrodynamic. And the proper weight distribution will help you avoid falling during pregnancy. Aim to keep your board flat on the water and your weight in the center. The board shouldn't nosedive and you should be flexible enough to step toward the tail when the wind picks up.

You can and should take breaks on the water. In the first trimester, your pregnancy won't be visible, but you'll feel the symptoms all right: you may be winded hauling up your sail or exhausted after a few runs. So when you need to take a break, know how to stop. Gently allow the rig to fall into the water, then squat and sit down on your board or take a quick dip to cool off and rest.

Cooling Down

After a good hour on the water, you'll need to stretch those tired muscles and drink a lot of water. After landing, secure your board and go for a little cooldown swim. This will help stretch out your arm muscles and allow you to do some flexibility work afterward while the muscles are warm. Focus on your arms and back. This part of your windsurfing workout is one of the most beneficial for your fitness. It will also help prevent backaches down the road.

Equipment Considerations

Your cherished windsurfing gear will serve you well during the first months of pregnancy—if you choose to take it out at all. I recommend working with gear that you are familiar with and very comfortable using. But if you're an advanced surfer and usually use a small board for high speed and jumps, you'll need to temporarily downgrade. You'll need to stick to Force 3 conditions or less—a smaller funboard needs Force 4 or above to sail and a sinker relies on Force 5 or greater wind. Choose a sail to correspond to your board and to the wind conditions. Don't experiment with new or more advanced equipment during pregnancy.

windsurfing

Other than your board, all you need is a good wetsuit, even in warm weather. A wetsuit will protect you from the sun, give you a little extra flotation when you're in the water, and prevent heat loss. Being cold will give you muscle cramps and isn't all that good for your circulation either. Since your belly isn't an issue yet, choose your suit in accordance with the water and air temperature. If it's warm, try a short-sleeved "shortie" or sleeveless "long john" wetsuit, for maximum arm flexibility. If it's very warm, wear at least a t-shirt to protect your body from the relentless UV exposure and prevent a bad sunburn.

Preparing for Difficult Situations

Windsurfing is only safe during pregnancy if you choose mellow, familiar conditions. This means avoiding areas with rocks, shallow reefs, currents, and cold water, and absolutely no windsurfing in dry-suit conditions (very cold water). And avoid waves. Consult the lifeguard and talk to the incoming windsurfers about the conditions. Even a familiar site can be very different—and unsafe for you when you're expecting—if the wind is inconsistent, an offshore wind is blowing, or the wind has whipped up some waves.

You have to take some common-sense precautions to be safe. First, windsurf flat water. Don't do any surf sailing, wave sailing, or jumping. Second, make ten knots (nautical miles per hour) your maximum wind speed. On the Beauford scale, this means you are looking for conditions between Force 0 (calm wind with a mirrorlike sea) and Force 3 (a gentle breeze at seven to ten knots with large wavelets). Avoid offshore winds, which will force you to struggle to get back to shore when you may already be worn out. Just call up the local weather center or check a local windsurf site for these weather details. Third, leave the harness at home. You won't need it if you are picking your conditions cautiously, and it isn't safe to wear during pregnancy because of the pressure it puts on your upper abdomen and back. Fourth, take breaks. You are exposed to a lot of sun out there and are working hard, so you need to get off your board frequently, rest, and, most important, hydrate.

Planning Pointers for Pregnancy

1 Be honest about your skill level. If you're a stable, regular windsurfer who can maneuver confidently and who just doesn't wipe out, you can make windsurfing a part of your early-pregnancy fun and games. If you're an occasional windsurfer with a lot of enthusiasm but less skill, hold off until after pregnancy, when those falls and tangles with your equipment won't be as risky.

2 Don't show off. It's tempting to try a few showy moves when you're feeling confident and the conditions are right. Hold back. Jumping, ripping, and racing can really get you into trouble and are not worth the risk during pregnancy.

3 Windsurf in straightforward conditions. Go out when there is a gentle wind and little, little waves (Force 0 to Force 3 conditions) with no offshore wind. Don't do any wave sailing or jumping. And avoid shores with rocks and shallow reefs, which could make your injuries even worse.

4 Choose your equipment conservatively. You'll still have a great time on the water if you're enjoying some easy sailing on a bigger board and can stop, float, and take a breather every once in a while. A sinker just won't let you do that.

5 Take breaks. Although you're not out of breath, you are using your muscles and will get tired. And you'll certainly get more worn out during pregnancy. So drop your sail and take a break, even while you're out on the water. Let go, stretch, and assess your energy level. If you're starting to tire or feel hot, head in for a longer break and a lot of water.

windsurfing

6 Test the water. Ideally, the water temperature should be between 82°F and 86°F (28°C and 30°C). If it's any warmer than that, you could overheat. On the other hand, even if it's a beautiful warm day, the water may be cool, requiring a wetsuit, which provides warmth, buoyancy, and serious sun protection.

7 Fall safely. When you begin to lose control and are about to wipe out, protect yourself from your equipment. Let go of your boom so your sail doesn't land on top of you. Try directing your fall so that you minimize the impact on your belly and vagina (feet first with your legs together, for example).

8 Hop in. Taking breaks in the water is really good for you during pregnancy. Swimming and treading water give you a bit of aerobic exercise, get your legs moving, and improve overall blood flow to your fetus.

9 Watch the sun. One of your greatest dangers on the water during pregnancy is the sun. Plan ahead to avoid sunburn and dehydration. Drink a lot of water ahead of time and go in frequently to hydrate. Wear a wetsuit or at least a t-shirt. And reapply lots of SPF-30 waterproof sunscreen every time you towel off.

10 Make windsurfing the highlight. Include walking or swimming in your exercise program so that you condition your heart and lungs too. It'll make you a stronger windsurfer and put you in great shape for the rest of your pregnancy and delivery. Plus, walking and swimming are activities you can enjoy right up until you give birth—and with your newborn baby, too.

surfing

There is a rhythm to catching waves that puts surfers in harmony with the ocean. Floating on the swell at sunset waiting for a last wave to take you in to shore is both meditative and thrilling. It's no wonder that surfers want to keep it up during pregnancy. If you are an experienced and confident surfer, you can surf safely through early pregnancy only—in low and uncrowded surf. No matter how ideal the surf, do not "get barreled" ("ride a tube") during pregnancy.

Surfing is excellent exercise—as you know if you've ever tried to swim straight out in the ocean and race the waves back in. You have to be a strong swimmer to paddle out, let alone to catch a wave. But simply being in the water is good for your pregnancy. As surfers know best, you can let the ocean do some of the work for you. The water helps support your weight, is easy on your joints, relieves ankle swelling, and keeps you cool. Plus, you can really work up an appetite out on the water, which will help you overcome that early-pregnancy nausea and encourage you to get the balanced diet you need.

If you are a strong and flexible surfer, you won't have trouble your first trimester when lying on your belly—your fetus is tucked behind your pubic bone and can handle the pressure. However, you do need to watch out for a couple of things, one from above and one from below. First, avoid getting too much sun. Second, avoid situations where you may get held underwater. You don't want to have to hold your breath during pregnancy—it can divert blood flow away from your uterus. As long as you surf conservatively, you can get some valuable exercise and stay safe.

Pregnancy is not a good time to learn how to surf, however. Paddling out is extremely strenuous exercise, since you are swimming against the waves, using only your arms. Even if the waves are small, you have to battle through the entire impact zone before you can even think about surfing. Waves can be fun and exciting, but they can also pound you if you are not perpendicular to the surf, are unprepared, are distracted, don't have control of your board, or just don't know what you are doing. And that's just half the challenge. Once you're out there, paddling to catch a wave is essentially a swimming sprint. If you aren't in top condition, it will just wear you out—and this isn't any good for your fetus, either.

As you can probably imagine, by your second trimester, your growing belly makes paddling out and popping up more of a challenge. Lying on your belly puts a lot of pressure on your uterus; women who have surfed in their second trimester report that they can feel their fetus move in relation to the board as well. Surfing is more risky after your third month because your fetus is vulnerable to injury if your board slams into you or if you are catapulted onto the water, which can feel like concrete if you hit it wrong. For this reason, I don't recommend surfing after your first trimester.

If you feel confident enough to surf early in pregnancy, just work on perfecting your form. In other words, surf in safe conditions where you can handle the waves with ease. Fear and ambition are what often generate the thrill of surfing: catching a big wave, riding an undiscovered break, and pushing your limits. But during pregnancy thrills like these should be avoided. Just as it does on land, this means moving cautiously and maintaining your balance.

If you are lucky enough to live in a town with warm water and gentle waves nearby, surfing can remain a staple of your exercise regimen your first trimester. I recommend mixing it up with some walking and hiking so that you are also doing some weight-bearing exercise to build your bones and prepare you for labor and delivery down the road.

RISK ASSESSMENT BY TRIMESTER

1ST TRIMESTER: MEDIUM
2ND TRIMESTER: HIGH
3RD TRIMESTER: HIGH

Staying Healthy Each Trimester

1ST TRIMESTER | RISK: MEDIUM

Surfing is only safe for experienced surfers this trimester. If you're still getting the hang of popping up on the board or have struggled with getting enough speed to catch a wave, then surfing is a bit too strenuous for you during pregnancy. You wouldn't want to risk a bad fall, potentially forcing water into your vagina and cervix (possibly causing a uterine infection) or simply hitting your head. Those perfect waves will be right there calling to you after delivery.

If you decide that you're experienced enough to handle a bit of surfing, pick a familiar beach where the waves are well below your usual level. Check the water temperature (the lifeguards may know) to make sure it is between 82°F and 86°F (28°C and 30°C). Water that is any warmer than that isn't good for your fetus—you could easily become overheated. If it's any cooler, and you should consider wearing a wetsuit.

Take care to not overexert yourself. Enjoy the water. Take breaks beyond the impact zone. Hang out on your board. And don't stay out longer than an hour; you need to come in to hydrate and reapply sunscreen to your delicate skin. Snack often—healthy foods like fruit will ward off nausea on the water.

Urinating a lot in the water doesn't necessarily mean you're well hydrated. It just means you're getting rid of some retained water. Being immersed in the water causes the extra fluid in your ankles, feet, and other tissues to return to your bloodstream, increasing your blood flow and keeping your blood pressure down, even while you are exercising. This is good for you—but you still need to drink plenty of water.

Surf as often as you can each week—and as often as the tide is right—for an hour each time. Walk on the other days to maintain your bone strength. After this trimester, try swimming or kayaking to maintain your strength and stamina. You'll be in fantastic shape, have fewer aches and pains, and enjoy a great attitude being on the water, where you want to be.

2ND TRIMESTER | RISK: HIGH

Your fetus is right there in front of you at this point and is vulnerable to all your falls, dives, and exertion. At this point in pregnancy, simply lying on your belly is not comfortable—or recommended. And diving is not a good idea either, because of the direct trauma to your belly. Play it safe and choose another fun water activity this trimester.

3RD TRIMESTER | RISK: HIGH

I'd be surprised if you even considered climbing onto a surfboard this trimester, when you can hardly reach your ankle to strap on the leash! Do some swimming and water aerobics to keep up your stamina and to reap the benefits of being in the water—but stay away from waves.

Since I run a surf shop in Santa Cruz, hitting the waves is part of my daily life. Of course, during both my pregnancies, I do think that I was more cautious on the water, but what surprised me was my husband's reaction. My husband, Ward, has always been supportive of my surfing. But I did notice that he was surfing with me more than usual once I got pregnant. I realized when he started calling people off waves that he was being protective. I can remember our midwife joking that she thought I should consider stopping because she was worried about the stress getting to Ward!

I could have kept surfing longer, but I knew that my center of gravity was changing and, although my balance seemed fine, I didn't want to risk falling on my board or getting pounded. So I just stopped standing up to ride. Up to about seven months, I could still take my board out and knee paddle, just crouching on my knees and paddling into calm water for the exercise. It was always nice to be in the water even after I stopped surfing—the buoyancy feels great when you're carrying those extra pounds.

Surfing really helped me with labor, too. My midwife said that surfers are good at working through labor because contractions are like waves. They grow stronger and stronger and then break. And there's a rhythm to them. Once I felt that, I was able to relax and go with the contractions instead of fighting them.

There are a lot of women surfers in Santa Cruz, including moms. One of my best friends also has a three-year-old son and it's great to be able to do beach days together. We take turns playing with the kids and surfing.

—Susan, Santa Cruz, California

Warming Up

Just carrying your board from the car or the rental shop has probably gotten your heart rate up and your muscles warm. While you're still warm, but before heading into the water, stick your board in the sand and do some stretching. Try dynamic stretches that target the shoulders, arms, neck, and back (see chapter 6). Then walk into the water to test the temperature. Go in up to your waist before climbing on and slowly paddling out, stretching your arms with each stroke.

Surfing Technique for Pregnancy

Paddling out will give you a great workout. Protect your belly and your balance by aiming right into the waves and lifting up slightly onto your arms to allow white water to pass around you while keeping your head above water. Once you're outside the impact zone, rest. You'll be winded and warmer than usual. This is not because you are out of shape—your body is surfing for two and paddling is intense aerobic exercise.

Your main concern while surfing during pregnancy is to be extra cautious about protecting yourself from injury. For example, if you don't feel the leash tugging at your ankle, cover your head with your arms when you resurface. Don't dive when you wipe out, just lean into the water so you don't accidentally encounter a sandbar headfirst. Pick an area that has few other surfers so you reduce your risk of accidents—and don't catch a wave with anybody. Introduce yourself to the surfers around you, so they are more likely to give you right-of-way. Enjoy gentle rides. Take breaks.

As you gain weight and your center of gravity gradually shifts, you will have to adjust your stance to center your weight so you don't "pearl" (nose-dive) or stall with too much weight on the back of the board. Surfing during your first trimester will get you in great shape to stay active during the rest of your pregnancy by conditioning your heart and lungs—and building your upper body and abdominal muscles.

Cooling Down

After you ride that last long wave to shore and carry your board in, take a few minutes to stretch the muscles you have been working so hard in the water. You can do some valuable stretching even while you're sitting on top of your board. Try stretching your arms to prevent soreness and stay limber. Once on shore, you can do some cooldown stretches to increase your flexibility (see chapter 7).

Equipment Considerations

You won't need to make many adjustments to your surfing equipment, since you won't be surfing beyond your first trimester, when your pregnancy isn't really visible yet and won't get in your way. But I will offer a few recommendations. You are going to get worn out more quickly out there and you need to take some breaks between waves. Consider using a board below your level (bigger, thicker, and uglier) so you have more flotation, can paddle with less drag, and can sit and rest on it.

Wear a wetsuit. There are a few good reasons to go to the trouble, especially during pregnancy. First, the suit will help you stay warm. Second, it will give you lots of extra buoyancy, so you can give your muscles a break. Third, it provides excellent protection from the constant UV rays on the water. And fourth, nothing makes you look like a fine surfing argonaut like a slick wetsuit.

If you're surfing in a swimsuit, you need one that is snug enough to stay put with every big wave. You just don't have time to make bikini adjustments when you're paddling. Pick a one-piece that supports your growing breasts underwater and out.

Preparing for Difficult Situations

Pregnancy is not the time to chase surfing challenges. Avoid areas with strong currents or reefs below the water. Check the tide tables ahead of time, consult the beach lifeguard, and talk to the incoming surfers about the conditions. A placid, calm break can be a different world when the wind, swell, and sea conditions change.

Planning Pointers for Pregnancy

1 Be honest about your skill level. If you are an experienced surfer and get out on the water regularly, you should be safe surfing during your first trimester only. If you are a beginning or occasional surfer, surfing may be too strenuous for you during pregnancy.

2 Stick to a familiar surf spot. The better you know the area, the safer you'll be. You'll know the sand bars, rip tides, reef breaks, and rocks. And you'll know where you can catch some small, reliable waves. Stay away from unfamiliar, empty, or rocky breaks. Beware of overconfidence when you're on vacation— if you are just visiting, try binocular surfing instead.

3 Take breaks. As all surfers know, you don't have to paddle all the way in to get a break. Just rest on your board in the lineup and wait for the perfect wave. Make sure you stop to catch your breath after paddling out so that you don't overexert yourself.

4 Underboard and overgear. Consider using a board *below* your skill level so that you have more flotation and can really sit on it when you're riding the swell. And gear *up*: wear a wetsuit if the water temperature isn't truly warm— it should be between 82°F and 86°F (28°C and 30°C) for warmth, buoyancy, and sun protection.

surfing

5 Fall safely. Rather than jumping or diving into the water when it feels like you might wipe out, lean into the water so that you minimize the impact to your belly and vagina as much as possible. If you don't feel the leash tugging your ankle, protect your head with your arms as you resurface.

6 Relax. Paddle in long, easy strokes and rest to stretch those muscles once you get past the impact zone. Breathe regularly and don't hold your breath longer than it takes to get through a short blast of white water.

7 Protect yourself from the sun. You are very vulnerable to severe sunburn while you're on your board. The best protection is a wetsuit; the next best thing is a long-sleeved t-shirt. And reapply a liberal coat of SPF-30 waterproof sunscreen every time you towel off.

8 Enjoy the Zen of surfing. If you are a confident surfer, you can enjoy dawn on the water, waiting for the perfect waves while watching the sun rise. The gentle, ever-present pull of the ocean propels your surfboard and it also promotes a positive lifestyle. There is something about surfing that makes you more even-keeled and optimistic. It's a healthy way to stay fit during early pregnancy—and to prepare yourself psychologically for the challenges and rewards ahead.

water skiing

Water skiing is a graceful sport that requires balance and speed. There really isn't a slow or easy way to water ski—once that boat powers up, you're on your way and there's no turning back. Water skiing is very risky during pregnancy. Why? You can fall with incredible force onto your belly, you can't control your speed, and, if you do fall, water may be forced into your vagina at about fifteen miles per hour. So it's not fun for your uterus and it's potentially hazardous for your fetus.

Even if you are a born-and-bred champion water skier and can guarantee no falls and gentle landings only—if that were possible—don't even consider water skiing past your first trimester, when the risk of trauma to the growing, increasingly protuberant uterus becomes far greater. There are many other, safer water activities you can enjoy this summer instead.

If you love being on the water, try kayaking. Not enough speed? Try sailing. Or man the speedboat while others water ski. And if you want a great workout that will truly benefit your baby, just jump in and swim for half an hour. Your love of water will serve you well during pregnancy, since the water allows you to feel weightless, gives your tired muscles and joints a break, and reduces your swelling. Plus, it is so refreshing. Getting in the water regularly will make you feel great—and keep you in fine shape for a healthy delivery, quick recovery, and a rapid return to water skiing.

RISK ASSESSMENT BY TRIMESTER

> **1ST TRIMESTER: HIGH**
> **2ND TRIMESTER: HIGH**
> **3RD TRIMESTER: HIGH**

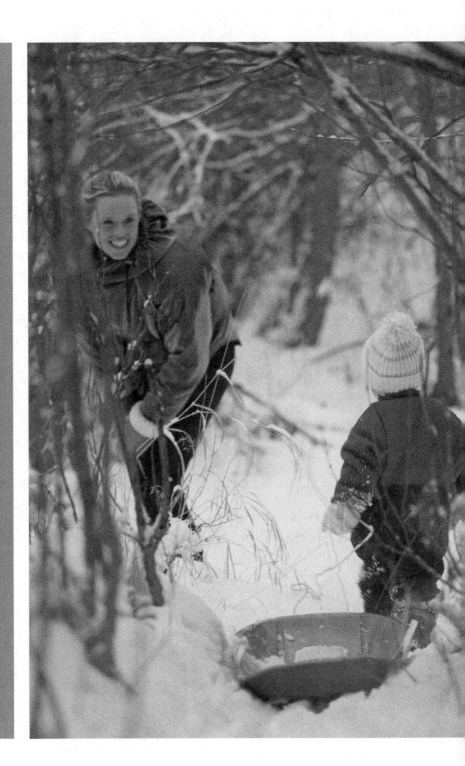

Staying Active on the Snow

Winter is the season when you are at greatest risk for feeling cooped up. It can be hard to leave that cozy fire, but there's a brilliant shimmering world out there waiting for you to explore it, even during pregnancy. Getting outdoors in the wintertime may be exactly what you need to beat the blues. Simply trudging into the snow is good exercise, but winter offers a host of other attractive and easy-to-learn options, like snowshoeing and cross-country skiing.

If you're a veteran skier or an impassioned snowboarder, you may be reluctant to give it up during pregnancy. You're not alone. One study published in the journal *Annals of Emergency Medicine* found that 2 percent of the skiers at a Colorado resort were pregnant. That's about one pregnant skier in every lift line! If the mountains are calling out to you this winter, just let caution be your guide.

Winter sports provide an excellent workout. Downhill skiing, snowboarding, cross-country skiing, and snowshoeing all work your entire body: arms, shoulders, back, legs, and abdomen. You'll find playing in the snow positively invigorating. If you're staying active this winter, your fetus will appreciate it too and may even feel the rhythm of your moving through the snow inside your uterus.

downhill skiing

Your winter may just not feel the same if you don't experience the anticipation, serenity, and rush of heading to the mountains for some downhill skiing. There's nothing quite like it. After all, gliding downhill captures a sense of freedom that is breathtaking—especially during pregnancy, when your body's changes may have you feeling cautious and downright clumsy. On the other hand, just the thought of becoming a parent may have done away with your passion for solo flight down a mountain. No? Then, read on.

Physicians have been understandably hesitant to condone skiing at all during pregnancy, in light of the steep slopes, the twists and turns, the temptation of greater speed, and the risk of flying out of control. But you're reading this book because you are careful and concerned—and eager to do the right thing for your developing fetus, even while you're dying to hit the slopes. If you're a veteran skier with years of experience, stable form, and confidence, go for it—but only during your first trimester.

The more stable and in control you are when you ski, the safer you are on the slopes. This means skiing a level or two below your skills. If you are an advanced stunt-woman (skiing black-diamond or double-diamond runs), you should downgrade to the intermediate slopes and "cruiser" runs. If you are a confident intermediate, ski the easy runs (blue squares) and beginner (green circles) slopes. Use your common sense to ski as smoothly as possible: no jumps and no moguls, since those quick turns and bumps are a real strain on your heart and muscles and are much more likely to cause falls. The conditions should be just right too, with groomed powder without patches of ice or rock and clear visibility.

Caution is your best guide, but here's the bottom line: a minor wipeout during the first three months of pregnancy should not cause a miscarriage, because your fetus is protected behind your pubic bone during your first trimester. During your second and third trimesters, however, a fall could indeed endanger your pregnancy; your belly is noticeably bigger and your fetus is more vulnerable if you fall—even if you don't land directly on your belly. Plus, as you hit bumps and hills, your knees compress into your belly, putting tremendous direct pressure on your uterus. That's why I don't recommend skiing at all after your first twelve to sixteen weeks.

Pregnancy relaxes your joints, ramps up your cardiovascular workout, and shifts your balance—all in the first few months. If you're not an experienced skier, these subtle changes can make you less stable, more tired, and vulnerable to injuries and overexertion. If you're a beginner or occasional skier, stick to flat ground during pregnancy—on cross-country skis or snowshoes.

And what about the altitude? Most ski resorts are well below the pregnancy danger zone of ten thousand feet. Besides, you'll only be at the summit for a few minutes anyway. Most resorts peak at around seven to eight thousand feet, a safe altitude if you have taken a few days to acclimatize, and the summit altitude should be posted at the bottom of the lift. A brief exposure (less than half an hour or so) to an altitude of over eight thousand feet as you get off the lift and make your way downhill should be safe for your fetus too. Confirm the altitude with the ski patrol before you head up the mountain and go back down right away if you feel unwell. Remember that you are more susceptible to altitude illness during pregnancy. If you're coming from near sea level, take a few days at lower altitude, at the lodge, for example, before you start exerting yourself.

Skiing is fantastic exercise. Not only do you burn an incredible number of calories carving down the mountain, but you also work the muscles in your legs, back, abdominals, and arms. Skiers are toned all over because skiing requires such balance, strength, and physical control. But it's also very tough on your joints, something you have to watch out for during pregnancy. Although having a ski on each foot helps you balance when gliding, you rarely have both skis on the snow when you're turning—and you're more likely to lose your balance and injure your knees or hips. So choose a good line down the mountain, avoid crowded slopes, and ski smooth and steady.

Skiing may feel like a tremendous break from pregnancy, but it really builds your muscles and stamina and works your heart and lungs for a more healthy— and pain-free—pregnancy. It is conceivable that your growing fetus may even feel the rhythm of your swooshing downhill. But your passion for the mountains and your desire to simply get outside (and stay fit for next season) will help motivate you to stay active during the rest of your pregnancy too—even when downhill is off-limits.

RISK ASSESSMENT BY TRIMESTER

1ST TRIMESTER: MEDIUM

2ND TRIMESTER: HIGH

3RD TRIMESTER: HIGH

downhill skiing

Staying Healthy Each Trimester

1ST TRIMESTER | RISK: MEDIUM

Skiing this trimester is only safe for experienced and confident downhill skiers. This is no time to learn to ski: experimenting with gear, hesitating about your turns, backtracking uphill to get on safe ground, heading down the mountain in a big wedge, or losing control from hitting an unexpected bump in the snow can all cause you to fall which is not good for your pregnancy. Overexertion with strenuous activity is worse. And skiing puts you at risk for both if you're not already a strong, fit skier.

No matter what your skill level is, forget the advanced slopes altogether—no black diamonds until after delivery. Stick to comfortable runs and move smoothly from one fall line (or turn) to the next. Choice slopes are groomed, covered in packed powder, and hazard free. That means no narrow valleys, no under-the-lift runs, and no going off piste. You'll still enjoy the mountains without that taste of danger.

You'll have to adjust your agenda according to your body's needs too. You'll be surprised to find that you've become out of breath, sweaty, and exhausted early on—that's normal: it's your pregnancy talking. Take breaks at the lodge or at the bottom of the slope, watching the experts fly down a slalom. Catch your breath, cool off or warm up as needed, and chug a lot of water. And make some relaxing plans for the late afternoon—like a fireside snooze.

Plan on being on the slopes for an hour at a time. Then, get out of the cold, take off your ski boots, and put your legs up for at least fifteen minutes—or however long it takes to drink a hot chocolate or herb tea. Assess how you feel and decide if you're up for another ski session. If you're starting to feel a little worn out, quit early: this is when you are most likely to tumble.

2ND TRIMESTER | RISK: HIGH

You've heard the stories of women who skied until they couldn't reach down over their big bellies to secure their own bindings. Yes, big pregnant women are out on the slopes all right, but I don't suggest that you join them. That big belly is your fetus right there in front of you. And he's no longer all that protected. Although you may have more energy this trimester, your balance is off—and is

"

We took several ski trips with friends when I was pregnant. With the slopes less than an hour away, we even slipped in some skiing on weekdays, when the runs were sublime. Long day trips were fun and exhilarating, but I noticed that I just couldn't move as fast as I did before the pregnancy. Or maybe I was just trying to ski in control rather than abandon myself to daredevil speed.

But I was surprised by how much I could do and by how good it felt to get outdoors. I thought I would end up hurting and tired, but the opposite was true. I felt rejuvenated and less sore after exercising. I was alert and refreshed both during and afterward.

Skiing with my friends kept my spirits up and made me feel like I was in control of my body, instead of feeling like the pregnancy was taking over and making me stationary and listless. For me, skiing was a positive way to stay in touch with others and socialize, rather than feel left out and cooped up in the house.

—Thuy, Denver, Colorado

"

constantly shifting, as your belly grows and as your fetus somersaults. Bumps on the slopes mean waves inside the uterus: your fetus feels every single one. And unexpectedly hitting a mogul might force your knees to slam into your belly, which is painful and could be dangerous.

If you are a very confident skier, you may not be able to resist skiing in the early part of this trimester, while your belly is still relatively small. But think about the many factors on the slopes you can't control, even if you yourself are in control—like ice or reckless skiers. At this point, even a mild slide onto your side would jolt your uterus and yank at your placenta. A tumble downhill could endanger your pregnancy. I recommend you stow your skis after about sixteen weeks, when trauma becomes a common cause of miscarriage.

Don't pass up that trip to the mountains, however: a traverse on back-country trails (in hiking boots, snow shoes, or cross-country skis) is a real thrill, too—and a much healthier activity for your fetus.

3RD TRIMESTER | RISK: HIGH

Sure, the mountains are filled with lovely scenery, but they're best enjoyed from a deck table at the chalet—ideally with your feet propped up on the bench in front of you. If the walk around the ski resort wasn't enough to get your heart pumping, lace on some snowshoes and give that powder a shot.

Warming Up

It's temping to just step into your bindings and head straight for the lift, but it's also a sure way to end up tired, sore, and possibly injured at the end of the day. If you're already in your skis, you can still warm up. In fact, your skis will give you some extra resistance. First, get your heart rate up for five minutes, either by trudging around in your boots to and from the car or by skiing some flat ground near the lift. Then activate the muscles you are going to use while skiing by standing in place and alternately lifting each knee toward your chest. Repeat five times on each side. Then plant your ski poles and gently jump, lifting both skis up so they remain parallel to the snow. Repeat ten times. Drop your poles and clasp your hands behind your head. Bend your knee and lift it up, reaching your elbow toward the opposite knee, stretching your back and abdominals. (You can also do these exercises at the top of the mountain, if you're getting cold and cramped.) Once you're warm, do some stretching to release your hips, arms, shoulders, and neck. Then head up for a couple very easy runs first, so you can get the hang of the skis and conditions.

Downhill Technique for Pregnancy

Your balance, control, and grace on skis depend on your stance. A neutral stance will allow you to respond quickly to an irregular surface, avoid unexpected obstacles, and keep your balance, which is fundamental to carving turns. Most important, it'll keep you from falling.

Your skis should be parallel, with your weight balanced over the center of your skis. Don't lean forward or sit back. Keep your ankles, knees, and hips balanced. As in good pregnancy standing posture, your pelvis should be tucked under you, so your abdominal muscles are firm. When you've got the stance right, you'll find that you can easily lift one ski off the ground completely. Sitting too low on your skis will tire you out much more quickly without improving your stability.

Although you can probably describe some of your most dramatic wipeouts in breathless detail, you've probably never given much thought to how you get up from that fall. Believe it or not, there is a right way to get up off the snow—especially during pregnancy when your back and joints are more vulnerable to injury. Rather than jerking yourself up using your back muscles, fueled by frustration, use the power of leverage. First, face your skis across the hill so you don't slide and end up in worse trouble. Then drive both poles into the snow just uphill of your hip. Put one hand on the baskets at the base and the other on the grips. Pushing into the poles with your arms, lift your body up over the tails of your skis until you are upright.

Cooling Down

After your last run of the day, cool down and stretch your tired muscles before you hop back in the car or head to the restaurant. Walk around the parking lot for five minutes to keep your muscles warm and get your blood flowing, especially to your hands and feet, which may be tingling. Stretch your arms, shoulders, back, and legs to minimize next-day soreness. If you find that your ankles swell up a bit after all those the hours in boots, elevate them above the level of your heart to get the blood circulating well.

downhill skiing

Equipment Considerations

Equipment can make or break your day on the slopes. I'm not just talking about your skis and boots; I mean your protective gear, too, down to your underwear. If you're cold and your muscles are tight, you're much more likely to become tired, sore, injured, and miserable.

Good skis and boots can certainly help you be a safer skier. No surprises here: during pregnancy, use familiar and comfortable skis. Experimenting with new gear is challenging since skis respond differently. If you're a traditional skier, stick to traditional skis. This is not the time to learn how to use telemark skis or deep side-cut skis (with somewhat of an hourglass shape) for carving.

You may opt for shorter skis for easier maneuverability during pregnancy. Also, a newer ski with greater longitudinal flexion, meaning it bends more easily, helps you avoid skidding during a turn and allows you to handle bumps and terrain more smoothly. Better performance materials give you more stability and control—just what you're looking for during pregnancy.

Comfort is also key, as are warmth and circulation. Wear layers so you are warm and dry, but well ventilated, so you don't get soaked with sweat. (You sweat more during pregnancy, even in the cold, because you are exerting yourself. Snowmelt is not the only way to have a soggy day.) Roomy, moisture-wicking long underwear is a good option, in polypropylene-based fabrics. You can even find panties and bras in breathable fabrics; fleece bras are an excellent option for preventing chafing against your tender breasts. Your two final layers should include a warm fleece or polypropylene pullover and a waterproof shell (ideally, with vents to allow ventilation.)

Pick boots with good arch support, but ones that aren't so tight that blood flow to your lower legs and feet is impaired—poor circulation increases your chances of frostnip. Make sure the wrist cuffs on your jacket aren't too tight, either—just cinched enough to keep the snow out. Thermal—not wool—socks, hat, and gloves also keep you warm and dry. And the warmer you are, the better your blood flow.

Your list of gear doesn't end there. Don't hit the slopes without sweat-proof sunscreen (SPF 30), lip balm, goggles, healthy snacks, and some water (a built-in water pouch in your backpack works well if you're not able to pause at the lodge for refills).

Preparing for Difficult Situations

Know your mountain. Safe skiing is a challenge, pregnant or not. But knowing what conditions to expect and planning cautiously is a big step in the right direction. Before you head up the mountain, make sure your ski resort is below ten thousand feet, a safe altitude during a healthy (nonsmoking) pregnancy.

What are the current conditions? Visibility, wind, temperature, and snow conditions are at least as important as your own skills on the slopes. The view may be spectacular, but you're also pretty vulnerable on the mountain. The resort's web cam is one way to see the mountain for yourself before you get there. Stay away from problematic conditions, like storms, fog, a poor base, and icy slopes. You're after groomed powder and groomed powder only.

Planning Pointers for Pregnancy

1 Ski confidently. Confidence and caution—not cockiness—keeps you safe on the slopes. Downhill skiing is a risky sport, with lots of variables and the potential for high-speed, high-impact accidents. If you are experienced and ski conservatively, you *can* be safe on the slopes—but you have to do everything you can to avoid falling and overexerting yourself. Ski well below your skill level and stay away from obstacles, crowded slopes, moguls, and catching air.

2 Learn after delivery. Pregnancy is not a time to learn to ski or practice your skills even if you're a stable beginner or a twice-a-year intermediate skier. Your body's already working overtime to support your growing pregnancy and getting worn out on the slopes just makes you more vulnerable to accidents.

3 Quit early. During the first twelve weeks or so of your pregnancy, your fetus is pretty well protected behind your pubic bone—and you're unlikely to endanger your pregnancy, even in a good tumble. After the early part of the second trimester, however, even moguls and minor falls can shake up your uterus, and a clumsy fall could cause real damage.

4 Work up to it. You have to be in good shape to ski downhill—it is an intensely cardiovascular and muscular exercise. If you are active (hiking, running, swimming) and have been skiing regularly, keep it up until the end of your first trimester. Your body will be able to handle it and you'll become even stronger and develop better stamina while skiing during early pregnancy. But don't hit the slopes if you haven't been there since last winter.

5 Suit up in comfortable gear. Fit, support, warmth, breathability, flexibility, and water repellency in your gear are key to safe skiing.

6 Practice good ski form. Proper posture on skis helps you ski better and helps strengthen the muscles you need every day during pregnancy, your lower back and legs. Bad posture—hunched shoulders, locked knees, an arched back—will wear you out faster and throw off your balance.

7 Fall safely and get up gracefully. Skiing in control, using every part of your body for better balance, allows you to anticipate your course and respond quickly to changes in terrain, unexpected bumps, and unpredictable skiers. If you do fall, use your poles and the gravity of the slope to help you up, rather than straining your back.

8 Go heavy on the sunscreen. The altitude, reflective snow, wind, and sun expose you to harsh UV rays that can really damage your sensitive skin. Slather on that sweat-proof SPF-30 sunscreen all over—and don't forget to protect the bottom of your nose, chin, and lips too.

9 Enjoy the ride, both up and down the mountain. Spending time on the snow is a real escape from the routines and rigors of daily life. A ski weekend is filled with heart-pumping exercise and social activities, but downhill skiing itself is also both meditative and intensely focused. On the lift, you experience a peacefulness that is rare at home.

snowboarding

Women have fallen in love with snowboarding, and for good reason: it's easy to learn, it's a sport with speed and grace, and it has a great community of hip, positive women. And there are pregnant boarders out there. Why? Well, first, there's something addictive about riding down a mountain. It's hard to pass up, even if you just got pregnant. And, second, for an experienced rider, snowboarding feels safer than downhill skiing in a couple of ways. Because you always have two feet planted on the ground, you have better balance, extra control, and more strength to use on each turn.

Your equipment can also make snowboarding a little easier during early pregnancy. New boards are so well designed that they have the flotation-like action of a surfboard combined with the versatility of an alpine ski. You can glide over powder or spring mush *and* carve down a mountain face. And unlike ski boots, which are hard plastic, snowboarding boots are more flexible and fully adjustable, so you can adjust your stance however you are most comfortable. In addition, you can get boots made just for women. Plus, having both feet attached to the board and basically immobile is easier on your hips, knees, and ankles—the joints most susceptible to injury during pregnancy. But, as with downhill skiing, the words to remember are *experience* and *caution.*

If you are a veteran snowboarder with several solid seasons under your belt and real confidence on the slopes, you can ride safely during early pregnancy. Ride well below your skill level. If you normally ride advanced slopes (black diamonds), ride intermediate (blue squares) instead. If you're usually on the intermediate slopes, stick to the beginner runs (green circles). Use your common sense to stay safe: no jumping, no moguls (bumpy ground is hard to balance on and pumping through those turns is exhausting), and no half-pipes. And stay away from ungroomed runs, icy slopes, and stormy conditions; good visibility and snow consistency help keep you safe.

Snowboarding is strenuous and the falls are hard on your body. If you're a beginner and you are a tad shaky, you consider falling to be the quickest way to slow down, and you still get a little panicky at the thought of getting off the chairlift, postpone your snowboard education until after delivery. Plus, being pregnant while snowboarding will simply wear you out—and make you even more likely to injure yourself. Ski flat ground instead and get a fantastic workout to show for it.

You may be concerned about going to a high altitude. After all, these are big mountains. Just make sure the highest run you plan to do is below the danger zone of ten thousand feet. Often, the altitude at the top is posted at the bottom of the lift where you get on. Most resorts are built at a safe altitude for pregnancy (usually below eight thousand feet), especially for short-term exposure. If the summit is above eight thousand feet, minimize your time up there. Even at a lower altitude, you are vulnerable to altitude illness and may need a day or two to adjust.

Snowboarding is excellent exercise—though it's so much fun that it doesn't feel like a workout. If you have a good stance, you'll have your stomach tucked in, with your belly firm and your back straight. As you burn through those turns, you're working your hamstrings, quadriceps, and glutes. When you push your edges into the snow, you're building your calves and smaller muscles up and down your legs. As you lean your weight back and forth, you build your abdominal muscles. And to keep your balance, you constantly adjust your arms to stay upright. If these skills have become second nature for you and you feel safe on the slopes, you can make snowboarding a highlight of your own winter games.

The stronger you become and the more practice you get, the better shape you're in for the rest of your pregnancy. Snowboarding builds back, legs, and belly muscles that you'll rely on as your uterus grows, and strength you'll use to push out your baby. If you're a riding junkie and you're not ready to give it up—just yet—go ahead and hit the slopes.

RISK ASSESSMENT BY TRIMESTER

1ST TRIMESTER: MEDIUM

2ND TRIMESTER: HIGH

3RD TRIMESTER: HIGH

Staying Healthy Each Trimester

1ST TRIMESTER | RISK: MEDIUM

Snowboarding is safe only for experienced riders this trimester. If you're a beginner (riding green-circle and occasional blue-square runs) or an occasional rider, your risk of taking a dangerous tumble are greater. At this point in your pregnancy, hitting your head is more of a risk than injuring the fetus, who is still protected behind your pubic bone. And even though your pregnancy isn't noticeable to others yet, you'll feel it as soon as you hit the slopes—you'll get sweaty, short of breath, and pooped much more quickly.

Pick comfortable, groomed slopes that you can cruise down and enjoy without falling. Let's be clear on one thing: a minor wipeout during the first three months of pregnancy should not cause a miscarriage; your fetus is protected at this point. But injuring yourself badly is more dangerous anytime in pregnancy. Choose a resort with a snowboarder-friendly attitude and uncrowded slopes. Steer clear of unfamiliar runs and obstacles; skip the powder between the trees or the run right under the lift. You're not after speed or air right now. Work on your stance and form instead.

Watch out for pushing yourself too hard. You can have such a ripping time on the slopes that you don't realize that you are exhausted and need to head home for a nap. Aim to take a sit-down break in the lounge every hour, even if you only make three runs in that time. You need to warm up and check in with yourself often throughout the day so you can give your body what it needs. Wear ventilated layers that you can peel off when you get hot. Plaster on that sweat-proof SPF-30 sunscreen. And hydrate, hydrate, hydrate.

2ND TRIMESTER | RISK: HIGH

It is no longer rare to see women with visible pregnancies on the slopes. I've heard plenty of stories of women who were on the slopes during their second trimester—even up to their sixth month. So yes, it can be done, but I still don't recommend it.

After about sixteen weeks, your growing fetus is more vulnerable if you fall—even if the impact is not directly to your belly. Your fetus is sitting right there in front of you and even a mild bump onto your behind causes a serious jolt to your uterus. Catching an edge and flying forward would cause a blow to your belly—and could put your pregnancy in jeopardy. Even an expert rider can't avoid all the risks on the mountain: an invisible patch of ice, a reckless skier, a ridge of hard-packed snow, or a beginner cutting unpredictable turns.

Your back is already under a lot of strain from carrying your increasing weight and your growing uterus. Maintaining a straight-backed snowboarding stance is a challenge when you're *not* pregnant, and it's a lot harder when you are.

It really started snowing my second month of pregnancy—dumping. My forty-year-old husband decided he was going to learn how to snowboard and I thought I'd show him how it's done.

Under the guise of giving him pointers and keeping him company, I went up with him, taking it slow and soaking in the scenery. The views of Lake Tahoe on that typical day were breathtaking. Easing myself through the powder was thrilling but peaceful too and just being up there restored my sense of self.

I'd been boarding for a good ten years and I'd almost forgotten about that brutal first day before the snowboarding mania kicks in. I believe my husband was in worse shape after a couple of hours than I was!

In the weeks that followed, we slipped in a little boarding between work and a few tremendous storms. And before you know it, he was raring to take on some bigger hills and I was deciding it was time for me to quit. I can't say why, but all of a sudden I didn't feel as comfortable on the slopes. I was very careful and I'd only fallen twice, but I was ready to stash the board until next year.

For the rest of the season, my husband hit the Sierras without me and I had to just listen to his stories of catching air and doing 360s. But, by that time, I could feel our baby moving and that was enough to take my breath away.

—Margaret, Lake Tahoe, California

snowboarding

Your body doesn't have its usual reserves to keep you strong and stable during a long, hard day on the slopes. Chances are, at a minimum you'd end up with a very sore back and a few days of recovery. It's not worth it for just a couple of hours of riding.

It's understandable that you can't resist the snow. Just strap on some cross-country skis or snowshoes and give your heart a pounding, instead of your body.

3RD TRIMESTER | RISK: HIGH

Take one look at your ballooning belly and you'll know you don't have the balance or flexibility to hit the slopes this trimester. And it's just too risky for your baby, who is right beneath the surface of your skin now. Do some hiking or snowshoeing to keep up your stamina on the snow—and you'll be set to hit the slopes next winter.

Warming Up

Once you lace up, you head straight for the summit lift, right? Think again. During pregnancy, you need to warm up your body slowly—it's very important for your developing fetus. Walk around a little first (especially if you just had a long drive up the mountain) to warm up your legs and get your heart going. Then do some dynamic stretches—you can do these even with your snow gear on—focusing on your hips, legs, and arms (see chapter 6). Squats and lunges will really prime those snowboarding muscles.

Then trudge over to the lift and do a few very easy runs to warm up your joints further and help you get comfortable with your board. You need to make sure your equipment is perfectly adjusted before you do anything else.

Snowboarding Technique for Pregnancy

The best way to stay safe on your board is to have a good stance. A neutral, or "ready," stance will allow you to be adaptable to changes in the snow (like a patch of powder or ice), be comfortable leaning into a turn, and protect your sensitive back muscles.

In the neutral stance, your knees are slightly bent, but your upper body is upright. Your hips and shoulders should be aligned as if you are sitting up straight in a chair. Your shoulders are relaxed, not hunched. As with good pregnancy posture, tuck your pelvis under you and squeeze your buttocks. Keeping your knees bent gives you more maneuverability and balance and keeps your center of gravity low to the ground, so you're less likely to fall. If you feel like you're losing your balance, don't straighten up—sink *lower* so you're more stable. Slam on the brakes by pushing down hard on your uphill edge.

During pregnancy, when your back is more vulnerable to injury and soreness and you weigh more, getting back up from the ground is a challenge. First, scoot forward so your bottom is as close to the board as it'll go. Press down with your heels so the board won't slide away from you. Then, grab the front edge to help you up to a squat. From there, use your legs, not your back, to stand up.

The most common snowboard injuries are those to the wrist, which occur when you reach back to break your fall. Wearing wrist guards can reduce your risk by half. Falling technique can help too. When you feel yourself falling, roll sideways and land on your hip, which is a more solid and wider surface than your wrist.

Cooling Down

After your last run of the day, cool down and stretch your tired muscles before you hop back in the car or head to the restaurant. Trudge around the parking lot for five minutes before you load your gear in the car. Stretching after riding will help you stay flexible for another day on the slopes and fight soreness. When you get back to your cabin or condo, get out of your boots and elevate your feet to take the pressure off your legs, preventing varicose veins and swelling later in pregnancy.

Equipment Considerations

Your equipment can do a lot for your technique on the slopes during pregnancy. Custom-fitted gear can make you more stable, less tired, better controlled, and more comfortable.

If you are usually a stable rider, but are having problems with balance or edging this time, the cause might be your gear; a little adjustment just might take care of those unsafe and awkward wobbles. Unbuckle or untie your boots, cinch them tighter, and secure your bindings so that your boots are firmly on the board.

snowboarding

Your boots are just as important as your board, especially during pregnancy. While you may want to consider using a longer board if you've gained a lot of weight, your boots will really keep you comfortable on the slopes. The essential ingredients include lightweight liners that fit your foot snugly; shock-absorbing soles to provide responsiveness and positive board feel; and waterproof, supportive shells. Even in the first trimester of pregnancy, your blood volume increases significantly, so good circulation is very important: if your feet are wet, uninsulated, unsupported, or constricted, you won't ride as well—or as long—and you may increase your risk of injury.

A helmet is another essential item on the slopes—your fetus's survival depends on your staying safe. More than 30 percent of boarders wear helmets, so you aren't alone, even if you feel silly wearing one. Look for a helmet with a snug fit and a lining that keeps you warm, since your head is where you lose the majority of your body heat.

Whether you're collecting meltwater on the lift or working up a sweat pumping down a slope, you need to stay dry. Wear layers of synthetic fabrics that keep you warm, ventilated, and dry on the inside and out. Since you sweat more than usual during pregnancy, start with roomy moisture-wicking undergarments made with polypropylene-based fabrics. On top of your warm fleece or polypropylene pullover, try a waterproof jacket with vents, so you can adjust temperature without having to pull off layers.

Pay attention to the little things, like good thermal socks, waterproof gloves, and underwear—those cotton undies will be soggy after a run or two. Bras, tank tops, and panties are all available in breathable fabrics, too. And some women swear by cozy fleece bras, which also help prevent chafing. Maintaining good circulation will decrease your chances of frostnip, so make sure those wrist and ankle cuffs are snug enough to keep snow out but are not constricting.

Right before you hit the slopes, cover your exposed skin with SPF-30 sweatproof sunscreen. Store lip balm with sunscreen in one pocket, some power snacks in another, and a bottle of water in your pack. Snap on your goggles and you're ready to go.

Preparing for Difficult Situations

Do a little research before heading to the slopes. Call the resort to find out what is this resort's top altitude. Almost all ski-resort summits are well below ten thousand feet—the majority are below eight thousand feet—and that's safe during a healthy (nonsmoking) pregnancy. If you're coming from sea level, however, take a day or two to adjust to the altitude before exerting yourself. Second, what's the weather going to be like up there? Remember, visibility and comfortable conditions are key to your riding safely. Third, how's the snow? Take a look at the resort's website and web cam for the most current snow conditions. You're looking for groomed powder—not icy patches or rocky outcroppings.

Before you go, prepare for intense UV exposure. The combination of sun, gleaming snow, wind, and high altitude are punishing to your extra-sensitive skin.

snowboarding

Planning Pointers for Pregnancy

1 Ride confidently. Snowboard during pregnancy only if you're an experienced rider, and only during the first trimester, when your fetus is better protected against falls.

2 Use caution. Stick to turf you know well and can practically ride with your eyes closed (or with the sun in your eyes). Ride a level below your skills. If you're a studly black-diamond (advanced) girl, choose the blue-square (intermediate) runs now. If you're a ripping intermediate, build your skills on green-circle (beginner) runs. Stay away from jumps, moguls, deep powder, slalom or obstacle runs, and ice. Choose slopes that aren't crowded, so you have stability, plenty of room to maneuver, and less risk of being cut off or bumped into.

3 Focus on good fit. Wearing snug, insulating, flexible clothing and gear is essential for safe riding. Comfort gives you confidence on the board. Take an extra five minutes to adjust your gear so that the fit is perfect—you'll be less tired, sore, and cranky and you'll be able to stay on the slopes an hour or two longer.

4 Helmet up. Helmets are a must on the slopes, especially given the unexpected tumbles you can take when boarding. Wear a helmet, even when you're taking it very easy, and keep your wits about you.

5 Take a break to watch the big girls ride. You can catch your breath (you'll be worn out sooner during pregnancy) at the side of the snowboard park or half-pipe while you take in the moves of the boarding royalty. Seeing how the really skilled boarders do it will keep you motivated to stay in shape during pregnancy, so you'll be ready to get back on the board after delivery. Catch your breath, cool off, give your tired muscles a rest, chomp on a snack, and hydrate.

6 Practice your stance. When you're expecting, boarding should be less about attitude and speed than it is about form and stability. Bent knees, a low center of gravity, and an upright back will keep you flexible and balanced—and less likely to wipe out or become intolerably sore.

7 Fall safely. If you have enough boarding experience to ride safely during the first few months of pregnancy, then you also have the savvy to protect yourself against injuries. If you begin to lose your balance, sink lower onto your board so you are even more stable. If you're going to fall, twist so that you land on your hip, rather than on your wrists.

8 Slop on the sunscreen. The altitude, reflective snow, wind, and sun will burn your face and lips if you don't protect yourself early and often. SPF-30 sweat-proof sunscreen and lip balm works well.

9 Remember: it's playtime. You should have a smile on your face. Take it easy, enjoy the scenery, and have fun. But if the conditions or your riding skills are making you nervous, head in.

cross-country skiing

In many ways, cross-country skiing is the perfect exercise. Although far surpassed in popularity by downhill skiing, cross-country skiing, also called Nordic skiing, is rapidly gaining fans. It's not just for star athletes and hardy wilderness explorers. Cross-country skiing is easy to learn and you can enjoy it right outside your doorstep (as long as there's snow). It's a great way to get outdoors in the winter, get in shape, and gather some peace of mind. Cross-country skiing is also a self-powered way to get around when the snow's too deep to drive in.

You may feel cooped up being pregnant in the middle of winter. But there's no need for you to hibernate in front of the fire. You will have more energy for the rest of pregnancy if you stay active. Cross-country skiing is a good solution. It's good for your growing fetus and it's really healthy for you.

If you are an experienced cross-country skier, you probably dusted off your skis the minute that perfect powder started falling. Cross-country skiing is a safe activity during pregnancy. If you've done it before, you already have the hang of the kick-and-glide stride and can handle the terrain. You're probably in pretty good shape, too; all that pumping with your legs and reaching with your arms gets your heart and lungs working and tones your entire body. You do have to choose your trails cautiously, though, and plan for shorter distances so you can take breaks and slow down when you get out of breath.

Falling is an unavoidable part of skiing, whether downhill or cross-country. Unless the snow is very hard, you've gained too much speed on a downhill, or you're heading straight for a tree, falls rarely hurt you. But twelve weeks into your pregnancy, your fetus is bigger and is more vulnerable if you fall—even if you don't land on your belly. The solution is control: set a comfortable pace and ski cautiously—or simply stay off skis altogether. You want to avoid that face plant at all costs.

If you begin to feel light-headed, nauseous, short of breath, or tired all over, rest. Your heart, lungs, and muscles need more breaks, snacks, and water during pregnancy. Also, the altitude may be affecting you. Although most trails are safely below the eight-thousand-foot limit recommended for exercise during pregnancy, you'll feel the effects of altitude well below that, even at three or four thousand feet, especially if this is your first day or two up on the mountain. So take it easy those first couple of days, especially if you are coming from near sea level.

As you explore the wilderness, from glittering meadow to glassy pond, you're conditioning your heart and lungs and improving the long-term circulation to your fetus. Research has shown that your rhythmic, gliding motion is felt inside the uterus, too, so it's a special way to bond with your baby. Plus, you're strengthening the muscles you use the most during pregnancy and will rely on after delivery when carrying your child: your legs, back, and arms. Cross-country skiing is too exhilarating and peaceful to feel like exercise, but it gives you all the benefits of an aerobic and weight-bearing workout, preparing you well for a healthier, quicker, and less painful delivery. After you recover, you will even be able to take your baby skiing with you after delivery in a special pull-along sled.

RISK ASSESSMENT BY TRIMESTER

1ST TRIMESTER: LOW
2ND TRIMESTER: MEDIUM
3RD TRIMESTER: MEDIUM

Staying Healthy Each Trimester

1ST TRIMESTER | RISK: LOW

I encourage you to try cross-country skiing during early pregnancy because it is such good exercise and a refreshing change from watching TV or clinging to the treadmill. A half hour on those skis will give you a whole new perspective on winter—and the long months ahead.

Fatigue and nausea may lay you low this trimester and it may be challenging simply to maintain a regular routine. To keep yourself motivated, mix it up. Walking, hiking, and snowshoeing are great alternatives. Cross-country skiing may become an event for days where you have time and energy to drive to a great park to ski. Try the ski machine at the gym first to condition yourself and get the hang of moving your arms and legs together smoothly. (During your first trimester, the ski machine is an excellent alternative to a regular outdoor routine. If you can only get out on the weekend, for example, do a half-hour indoor ski workout a couple of times during the week to stay in shape. After your first trimester, however, your belly will get too big to comfortably lean against the hip or abdomen supports and balance can become difficult.)

cross-country skiing

When you get out on the trail, you are likely to become tired more quickly. It is normal to find yourself bathed in sweat and panting, despite the flat trail and near freezing temperatures. Slow and steady wins the race. Choose trails with little grade, no steep downhills, and no killer uphills. Your joints are more vulnerable to twists and sprains during pregnancy. And even though it is cold, you are losing fluids—all that sweating and panting—and you have to hydrate well. You're also burning a lot of calories, so nutritious snacks are a must on the trail.

Cross-country skiing is a sport you can learn during your first trimester. It requires coordination, agility, and stamina, but if you're up for it, give it a try. Cross-country skiing is a very natural movement, like gliding across the gym floor in socks, as you probably did when you were a kid. Start with a shuffling walk and slowly add more glide to each shuffle. You'll feel wobbly at first, but you've got both feet on the ground, the length of the ski to give you balance, and your poles to prop you up. With a little practice on a snowy golf course or parking lot, you will begin to feel more stable and ready to hit the trail. But use your common sense: stick to flat trails with lots of room to maneuver and few obstacles (for example, few trees and reckless skiers), and look for good visibility and snow consistency.

If you're a beginner, start with about half an hour of cross-country skiing; it may not sound like a lot, but it is plenty of exercise. If you're fit and experienced, make an hour your maximum on the trail. Once you get out on the snow this trimester, you may feel unstoppable. But make a point of getting out of the cold and snacking regularly.

2ND TRIMESTER | RISK: MEDIUM

If you are a confident cross-country skier and live near some good snow, you'll really enjoy your second trimester. Once the morning sickness is out of the way and your body has adjusted to being pregnant, you'll probably have lots of energy—and want to get outside. Go for it, as long as you're a veteran skier.

If you ski cautiously, you can prevent getting out of control and having a bad fall. But it can still happen. Although cross-country falls are less ugly than downhill tumbles, even a mild thump onto your side jolts your uterus. I therefore only recommend cross-country skiing after the first trimester to experienced skiers. Stability is key to safety at this point in pregnancy. (According to some women, though, your shifting center of gravity improves your balance on skis.)

"Cross-country skiing was an integral part of our lives before pregnancy. Heading out to the backcountry to ski was one of our special winter trips that I wasn't willing to sacrifice just because I was pregnant.

I found that I had to ski for shorter periods of time, as my level of stamina was not what it had been. But I was able to ski without pain, discomfort, or challenge. I found that mostly I needed to carry snacks and allow plenty of time for rest in the evening. Although we had wanted to stay in a backcountry yurt (a Mongolian ski hut) I was comfortable in a more traditional room in a lodge with a double bed, heated bathroom, and movies. It still enabled me to enjoy skiing, but it also helped me address the needs of my pregnant body and mind.

Staying active doing the things I love helped me deal with my changing body and growing stomach (which I had worked my whole life to keep flat). Being physically active also reduced my stress level and eased my concerns about the transition my husband and I were making to family life.

I realized that I could be pregnant and continue my favorite activities. Although I might need to make some adjustments, I know I won't have to sacrifice my love of outdoor activities and sports either before or after I become a mother.

—Kate, Ithaca, New York"

cross-country skiing

Skiing on groomed trails—also known as track skiing—is safest. First, maintained terrain is more predictable (less risk of falling through hidden ice into a creek, for example). Second, you can take a look at a map and choose the length and grade you feel comfortable with. Third, you are typically closer to help if you need it, and less likely to lose your way. Last but not least, they have convenient restrooms for that active bladder.

Avoid snowed-over roads and backcountry ski trails. You are likely to encounter deep powder and ice, which make falls more likely.

If you've been skiing or working out regularly, you should be able to ski for an hour at a time this trimester. Many women find that their stamina increases considerably after the sixth month, so this is a good time to ski with friends, or bond with your baby. As you ski, your baby may kick or nap, a sign that she is responding to the gentle rocking of your motion across the snow. The more active you are this trimester, the easier your third trimester will be and the better your attitude will be.

3RD TRIMESTER | RISK: MEDIUM

At this point in pregnancy, I recommend cross-country skiing only for women who are in excellent shape and have been on the trails regularly this pregnancy. If you're a beginner or occasional skier, the shifted balance caused by your big belly will really throw you off and even gentle falls are very risky, since your baby is right below the surface of your taut belly. Also, the relaxed ligaments in your pelvis, causing the characteristic pregnancy waddle, can make your stance on skis somewhat less stable than it was before.

If you're not up for skiing but want to stay in good shape, try rowing (kayaking or canoeing outdoors or using a rowing machine), which also works your upper and lower body simultaneously and doesn't carry the same risk of injury. Hiking and snowshoeing are also fantastic options, since you'll get good exercise while refreshing your mind in the wilderness.

Even a few minutes on the snow will give you a tremendous workout this trimester, since you are carrying extra weight and are working against the resistance of the snow. For this reason, it is especially important to warm up and cool down adequately. You may notice that this strenuous exercise stimulates Braxton Hicks contractions. Don't worry: these contractions should disappear after a few minutes of resting.

cross-country skiing

There is no cut-off date for cross-country skiing during pregnancy. Some active women who live in snow country make cross-country skiing a part of their daily routine until close to delivery. It's a great way to fight cabin fever, especially when the snowplow hasn't shown up. If you're very comfortable on skis and just don't fall, you can ski late into pregnancy. But if you develop back pain and fatigue easily, or if you find that your coordination isn't what it used to be, you may decide to turn in your skis during your second trimester or earlier. Good for you: you are the best judge of what feels safe.

Warming Up

Don't let your enthusiasm get the upper hand. Taking ten minutes to warm up now will prevent some serious soreness, exhaustion, and grumpiness down the trail. Bundle up, put on your boots, and trudge around near the trailhead to get your heart rate up. Then put on your skis and ski a flat surface, focusing on your form and the length of your glide—not your speed or progress.

Next, pause to do some dynamic stretching (see chapter 6). Try some squats and lunges, using a tree or railing for support. With your skis on, you can do some in-place exercises that improve blood flow—these are also useful if you're feeling cold or cramped on the trail. Stand with your skis parallel, then alternately lift each knee toward your chest. Repeat five times on each side. Then plant your ski poles and gently jump, lifting both skis off the ground, parallel to the snow. Repeat ten times. Drop your poles and clasp your hands behind your head. Bend your knee and lift it up, reaching your elbow toward the opposite knee, stretching your back and abdominals. Shoulder and arm circles will warm up your upper body so it can provide strong support using your poles. Head toward the trail and start soaking in that wondrous landscape.

Cross-Country Technique for Pregnancy

Before you hit the trails, you should have the basics under your belt and feel confident turning, slowing down, and stopping. If you want to learn these skills, take a lesson or two during your first trimester to get some expert tips and practice on easy, wide trails where you are not likely to fall. Good form on your skis is the same whether you are pregnant or not: your upper body is relaxed, your back slightly rounded, your arms swing from the shoulders, and you lean your weight

cross-country skiing

forward slightly at your ankles when you want to speed up. Use your poles for balance and to help propel you forward.

Keep your knees and ankles slightly bent so have some flexibility in your stance to handle bumps in the terrain and for better maneuverability. Keep your eyes on the trail about twelve feet in front of you—not on the tips of your skis, which will make you wobbly. As you glide, keep your weight centered on the weight-bearing ski, so that that ski doesn't tip sideways or suddenly dig into the snow.

If you're not feeling quite balanced, figure out why before you're too far from home base. Are you too tired to ski? Too cold and stiff? Do your boots need adjustment? They should feel tight and supportive. Are you maintaining a proper stance? If you're just not comfortable or feel unstable, head home before you get frustrated or hurt.

If you ski cautiously, you can anticipate your falls—and minimize the resulting damage. This technique is called "bailing out" and it allows you to take control of your fall *before* it slams you. Whether you trip on a rock or hit an icy patch on a downhill, if you start to lose control bend your knees and crouch so that you fall onto your side—somewhere between your buttocks and hip bone. Your flank is a soft, wide surface and will break your fall. After your first trimester, your fetus will certainly feel it, but it's a lot safer than falling onto your belly or tender tailbone.

From this position, you can easily stop sliding and safely get back up, even if you're on a hill. Roll onto your side, uncross your skis, and bend your knees, so you are in a fetal position. If you're on a hill, make sure your skis are facing across the slope. Use your hands to scoot your body into a squat above your skis. Take it slow, since you may become light-headed if you get up too quickly. Then slide one ski forward and stand up, using your poles for balance. This technique works a lot better than haphazardly trying to get divergent skis under you or trying to stand up from sitting on the tails of your skis as they conspire to shoot out from under you like icy rockets.

Remember to take breaks. Unlike downhill skiing, cross-country has no built-in breaks, such as waiting in the lift line or riding up to the summit, for you to catch your breath and cool off. Make sure you are stopping frequently to rest, snack, and hydrate.

Cooling Down

After all that rigorous exercise, your muscles will have built up their share of lactic acid—the natural chemical that causes cramps and soreness. A simple cooldown routine will help circulate some blood to those tired muscles and prevent aching the next day. After you catch your breath at the end of the trail, take ten minutes to take an easy ski around level ground. Once your heart rate is back down, stop and stretch those warm muscles. Focus your stretching on your arms, shoulders, back, and legs. You may find that your ankles swell up a bit when you get them out of those boots—put them up on a chair to get the blood circulating well again.

Equipment Considerations

You don't need any special equipment for cross-country skiing during pregnancy. Your typical light-touring skis, boots, and binding will work just fine. If you're a passionate downhill skier who has switched to cross-country for the duration of the winter because of your pregnancy, you'll find you're much more comfortable in this gear than in your downhill equipment. The boots are more flexible and lightly constructed than downhill boots. If you're renting or buying cross-country boots, look for boots that come up over your ankle to offer good support; these are called "combination" boots. Low-cut racing boots are lighter, but give little support, so avoid them during pregnancy.

Choosing skis during pregnancy is easy. Stick with the ski length you are usually comfortable with. The traditional or long skis will give you better balance and gliding ability since they don't sink into the snow as deeply, and the mid-length skis (about head height) are easier to turn and glide on packed snow. Since you're going to be on groomed trails during pregnancy, pick medium-width skis. Narrow skis are for racing and give you less help with balance, and wide skis won't fit as well into machine-groomed tracks (they're designed for going off trail). There is no right or left ski, so you can't go wrong once you've got your skis picked out.

You'll want step-in or automatic bindings, especially if you're skiing later in pregnancy, when bending over is uncomfortable and can make you lightheaded. Poles with a hoof basket are intended for groomed trails and round baskets are for loose powder, but both will work fine for light touring.

cross-country skiing

What you wear is key to your comfort on the trail. You are going to get hot, even though it's cold out, so you'll need less clothing than you would for snowshoeing or downhill skiing. Since you sweat more during pregnancy, especially when you're doing something as rigorous as cross-country skiing, the innermost layer is as important as the outermost. Layering allows you to fine-tune your clothing depending on the weather and the level of your workout. The layer nearest your skin should be moisture wicking, like polypropylene-based fabrics. On top of this, wear a bulkier fleece or wool layer for warmth, then a windproof and water-resistant shell. Pull your socks and gloves smooth so you maintain blood flow to your hands and feet, helping them stay warm and preventing blisters. Try wearing spandex cycling shorts instead of cotton underwear. These won't get soaked in sweat and they help prevent chafing.

You're just not ready to hit the trail until you're gussied up in your hat, gloves, a scarf or neck gaiter, and some UV-protective sunglasses. And if you want to avoid the "raccoon" look, slop on the SPF-30 sweat-proof sunscreen, even in cloudy weather, and especially if you're at altitude.

Preparing for Difficult Situations

Play it safe when choosing your cross-country route. Pick a park (whether it's a ski resort or national park with groomed cross-country trails or the local park with marked paths) with groomed snow and marked trails. Find out the highest elevation before you head out; it should be below eight thousand feet. Most resorts are comfortably below this altitude. If you're coming from near sea level, take a day or two to get used to the altitude. Stay away from mountaineering runs (climbing a mountain on skis), steep downhills, and crowded trails. Check up on the snow and weather conditions before you go: ice, wind, or rain could make you miserable, and poor visibility and snow consistency could impair your safety.

Planning Pointers for Pregnancy

1 Take it slow and steady. Cross-country skiing is a rigorous sport but safe enough to learn during the first couple of months of pregnancy if you're an athletic woman. Take the time to master the basics and don't push yourself. Take a lesson to help you feel stable and proficient at turning, slowing down, and stopping effectively. If you're already a cross-country buff, choose trails that give you a good workout without putting you at risk for falls and overexertion. And take breaks at least every hour to hydrate and cool down.

2 Train before you hit the trail. Cross-country skiing requires balance, strength, and stamina. Training off the snow will give you more confidence on skis. Practice on a ski machine indoors until you get the hang of it, or build your stamina during the off-season by rowing, hiking, or swimming.

3 Ski with caution. Pregnancy is not the time to fly willy-nilly downhill or venture off the track into the forest. You'll get the thrills of a different sort if you keep your eyes open on the trail, like when you see a moose scratching itself against a nearby pine. Staying on groomed tracks will help prevent falls (the track helps keep your skis parallel and heading the right direction) and encounters with unexpected obstacles.

4 Focus on form. Pregnancy is a great time to stick to really work on your kick and glide technique while sticking to easy trails. It's exhilarating to get into the rhythm of cross-country skiing and your baby in utero will probably enjoy it, too.

cross-country skiing

5   Layer for warmth and flexibility. Your clothing should wick moisture away from your skin and keep you dry in case it is snowing or raining—or in case you fall. More likely than not, you'll feel like you've been in a sauna after a quarter of an hour on the trail and will have to peel off a layer or two.

6   Fall safely. Skiing in a controlled manner and anticipating your falls will allow you to protect yourself and your pregnancy. If you feel unstable, bend your knees deeper to get your center of gravity closer to the ground. Bail out if you have to by falling sideways onto your flank. This protects your belly and your tender tailbone. Then, you'll be in a good position to get up without getting your skis tangled or sliding downhill.

7   Slather on the sunscreen. Your skin is more vulnerable to sun- and windburn during pregnancy and the reflective snow and altitude exposes you to lots of dangerous UV rays. The solution is to cover your exposed skin with a generous helping of SPF-30 sweat-proof sunscreen.

8   Listen to the silence. Despite being one of the most physically rigorous exercises you can enjoy during pregnancy, cross-country skiing is extremely meditative. As you glide through the hushed wilderness, the rhythm of your arms, legs, and breathing becomes almost effortless, and the tingle of crisp air on your skin vaporizes your stress. If getting on skis makes you nervous, go with your instincts and stick with something you can really enjoy instead. But if you're up for it, cross-country skiing will beat your winter blues and keep you in great shape for the rest of pregnancy, delivery, and parenthood.

snowshoeing

Showshoeing is quickly gaining in popularity and you'll see why the minute you strap on your snowshoes: it's as easy as walking and it makes the winter landscape your playground. You'll even start to think of a blizzard as something to look forward to. If you enjoy the exhilaration of hiking in the wilderness, exploring the same places on showshoes will blow you away. You'll find familiar places transformed by the luminescent snow and feel humbled in the awesome silence of the frozen mountains or prairie.

The ease of snowshoeing, the excellent exercise, and the peace of mind it nurtures make snowshoeing an ideal exercise choice during pregnancy. It may not have occurred to you as a pregnancy workout option. But that may be because you've been keeping cozy indoors ever since the sidewalks froze. But those conditions are perfect for snowshoeing.

A terrific aerobic exercise, snowshoeing works your heart and lungs, strengthens your muscles, builds stamina, and is pretty easy on your joints and back. Because it is also a weight-bearing exercise, it is good for your bones. After snowshoeing regularly, you'll be in fantastic shape for a healthier and quicker delivery. And compared to your other outdoor winter exercise options, like snowboarding, cross-country skiing, or downhill skiing, you are much less likely to fall or be injured; you also can enjoy snowshoeing a few times a week near home without having to get to or buy tickets for a resort.

Don't get me wrong: snowshoeing is not a cakewalk. It's intense exercise. Several factors make it a tougher workout than hiking. First of all, you slip a little with each step, so it's two steps forward and one slide back. Plus, with each step onto new snow, the snowshoe sinks in, which makes walking a flat trail feel like climbing stairs. On top of that, the cold will wear you out, since your body has to work to keep warm, and you must carry the weight of the snowshoes. Even though the new lightweight aluminum models don't weigh a lot, you'll certainly feel their weight when you have to lift your leg high to clear the snow with each step.

Heading deep into the backcountry, away from roads, snowmobiles, and even trails may be tempting, but it's not a safe plan during pregnancy. Instead, stick to established routes so you can pick gentle trails with fine views but also ski patrol personnel, nearby restrooms, and maps. I do not recommend

snowshoeing

mountaineering, ice climbing, using ropes or ice picks, traversing crevasses, or venturing off trail when you're expecting, even if you're in great shape. The key is to move gently.

Although the better snow and quieter trails may be more easily found in the mountains, the altitude there can also contribute to your exhaustion. To be safe, stay below eight thousand feet. If you're coming from near sea level, take at least a day or two to get used to higher altitude by staying below six thousand feet. Even at lower altitudes, you may feel unwell and short of breath. The solution is to rest, take a few relaxed days to get acclimatized and head down the mountain if you can.

Even if you just learned to snowshoe during your first trimester, you can enjoy the sport far into pregnancy. There is something magical about wandering through a glittering wonderland. It will get your spirits up in winter, when you may start to feel like a blob. Staying active will give you some control over your body, improve your moods, boost your energy, and get you in great shape for the rest of pregnancy, delivery—and recovery. If you've become a snowshoeing enthusiast, you'll be happy to know that you can bring your youngster with you as soon as he's old enough to ride in a backpack.

RISK ASSESSMENT BY TRIMESTER

1ST TRIMESTER: LOW
2ND TRIMESTER: LOW
3RD TRIMESTER: MEDIUM

Staying Healthy Each Trimester

1ST TRIMESTER | RISK: LOW

Even if you've never been on showshoes, you can learn this trimester. It does take some skill and balance, but you're not likely to fall and you can take it as slow as you like. Padding through powder is a lot easier and more fun than you'd expect— even if you're used to downhill skiing or playing fireside chess in the winter instead. If you've done a lot of hiking before, you'll get the hang of snowshoeing without delay. If you haven't spent much time on the snow, practice on wide, flat surfaces, like a park service road, and consider taking a lesson.

"Before I was pregnant, we would go hiking in all sorts of weather—here in Vancouver, you have to if you want to get outdoors. During pregnancy, I got pickier about the conditions. So, when the mountains were shining with snow and the sun made an appearance about halfway through my pregnancy, we couldn't resist trying snowshoeing.

I was slow—my husband told me I waddled. I had a fantastic time anyway. If I had realized how easy snowshoeing is, I would have tried it much earlier. Learning during pregnancy gave me a boost and reactivated my outdoor self.

The biggest challenge was fitting into my gear. They just don't make parkas and ski pants to fit over bellies like that and, even if they did, I wouldn't want to pay for it.

One thing I have since learned is that for snow sports, it's nice to stay close to home. I found that I felt overextended when we drove a long way to go snowshoeing. But when we stayed nearby, I could take breaks without feeling like I was missing out.

Now we own snowshoes and, by the way, they come in kids' sizes too.

—Anabel, Vancouver, Canada"

snowshoeing

In the first couple of weeks of pregnancy, your body experiences significant changes that may make you more tired, vulnerable to injury, and susceptible to dehydration and altitude illness. If you feel worn out or nauseous, develop a headache, or are short of breath, take a break and consider heading back. If it doesn't feel right to you, it isn't any good for your fetus, either.

No doubt you feel less energetic this trimester and are having difficulty maintaining a regular exercise routine; the advantage of snowshoeing is that it doesn't take a lot of preparation and equipment, if you live near some snow. On off days or weeks, mix it up with some hiking, biking, or even skiing. Some women find that any exercise in the crisp winter air reduces nausea and builds up a healthy appetite.

Watch out for pushing yourself too hard when snowshoeing—a strenuous path with deep powder or a mighty uphill will be rough on you and your fetus. You can overheat on the snow, so removing layers when you feel warm is important for keeping your temperature low enough for your fetus. Take breaks to assess your distance covered, munch, chat, and drink up—you're sweating and burning a lot more calories than you realize.

Aim for a half-hour excursion to start. Depending on the trail, you may cover less than half a mile. Once you get the hang of it, work up to snowshoeing for an hour a few times per week. Or, if you have to drive to the snow, save snowshoeing for weekend excursions and stay active in town with regular walks or gym workouts.

2ND TRIMESTER | RISK: LOW

Snowshoeing is also safe and healthy during your second trimester, even if you're a beginner. As always, exercise cautiously and listen to your body. If you've been active thus far in your pregnancy, chances are that you'll be able to tackle longer trails this trimester, with your nausea and fatigue out of the way. Your belly isn't quite big enough yet to throw off your balance, though you'll feel the increase in your weight and the strain in your back muscles; stretching en route is the solution.

To avoid injury to your back, carry only a light pack. To prevent ankle and knee injuries, since your joints are lax during pregnancy, always aim your foot in the same direction as your snowshoe. This may seem self-evident, but your bindings do allow some play and your feet may tend to splay out in the typical pregnancy waddle or even turn inward if they're tired. Remove collected snow from your shoes, dig in for traction with each step, and focus on stability to prevent falls, since your uterus is more vulnerable this trimester.

Believe it or not, going a half mile per hour is a fast pace. Plan to cover short distances (an hour at a time—including breaks on the trail) and flat terrain. Packed trails are easiest, since you are not breaking new snow. If you're in a group, let the most fit and energetic person take the lead, at least some of the time. Place your shoes in the footprints of the leader as much as possible, to conserve energy and create a well-defined trail for the way back. Stick to a comfortable, even pace, even if others in your party are running ahead or skidding down hills—pushing yourself too hard and possibly falling is just not worth it during pregnancy. Remember, your heart is pumping for two, so avoid extra exertion.

3RD TRIMESTER | RISK: MEDIUM

If you've been snowshoeing or hiking comfortably this pregnancy or are simply in excellent shape when the first snowstorm hits, you can head out for some gentle snowshoeing this trimester. Keep in mind that your big belly and forward-shifted center of gravity make you less stable on the trail and unable to see the track right in front of you. Be a careful judge of your abilities. If you feel confident on snowshoes, stick to flat, wide, even surfaces and groomed or packed snow. Lifting your knees high enough to blaze a trail across new powder is not feasible or fun. And you need to avoid a face-plant at all costs.

Snowshoeing is an attractive option late in pregnancy because of your ability to control your pace, get away from civilization even in grim weather, and use finesse rather than brute force to move. But this is rigorous exercise, so take it slow. And don't be surprised if you develop some Braxton Hicks contractions mid-route; these practice contractions are triggered by the exercise and will go away after you rest for a few minutes.

If snowshoeing is too tiring or makes you feel unstable this trimester, staying off the trails is a healthy decision. You should feel confident and have a smile on your face. If not, there are plenty of other enjoyable options, like hiking lower-elevation trails with no snow.

snowshoeing

Warming Up

Rigorous exercise like snowshoeing requires a good warm-up. Gradually activating your muscles will get your blood circulating to the organs that need it, like your heart and muscles, without suddenly decreasing blood flow to important internal organs, like your uterus. Plus, stepping out of your toasty house or car into near-freezing temperatures is a shock to your body and it needs a little time to adjust so it can maintain a healthy temperature.

Walking is the best warm-up for snowshoeing. There should be an area of firmly packed snow at the trailhead or around the parking area where you can trudge around for five to ten minutes to get your heart rate up. If you're surrounded by deep snow—let's say it just snowed a couple of feet last night and you plan to walk a quarter mile to the grocery store—put on the snowshoes and march in place for five minutes, bringing your knees high toward the chest, to stretch out your legs and get your blood pumping. Squats and lunges—with support—are also safe to do in boots or snowshoes.

Then pause for some dynamic stretching, focusing on your legs, hips, shoulders, and arms (see chapter 6). It will help to keep you limber and prevent cramps and soreness in those muscles the next day. When you get cold or stiff on the trail doing these stretches will help send extra blood to those muscles and keep you energized.

Snowshoeing Technique for Pregnancy

If you can walk, you'll be able to snowshoe. On modern aluminum snowshoes, you walk with a basically normal gait, so slowing down, turning, and stopping are instinctive movements. For the gently graded, packed trails you're going to be on during pregnancy, that's pretty much all you need to know. Certainly, many experts traverse steep slopes, climb a quick-frozen hard crust, handle ice, and even cross crevasses, but you're not going anywhere near those challenges right now—even if you've tackled them before.

Good posture will serve you well on snowshoes as well as off. If you keep your knees relaxed, your shoulders and hips aligned, your pelvis tucked under you, and your back straight, you'll feel less strain in your lower back and will be more stable on your feet. As your belly grows, your tendency is to arch your lower back and allow your belly to stick out, which thrusts your weight forward instead of squarely over your hips and throws you off balance. You can practice a healthy stance by looking at your profile in a mirror. Firm up your abdomen and buttocks and tuck your pelvis under. Notice how your back is straighter now. Keep that posture whether you're snowshoeing, hiking, or shopping.

You're working some less-used muscles here, even if you're an avid hiker, runner, or skier. Mainly, you're working your legs and arms, especially if you're using poles. But if you keep good posture you will also tone your back and abdominals. Depending on the snow conditions and your snowshoes, you may have a fairly normal gait, especially if you have a pair of modern snowshoes, with their streamlined, compact design. On older snowshoes, your legs are somewhat farther apart because of the width of the snowshoes, so you really work your inner thigh muscles. Turning, jumping, going up and down hills, and even running are easy to do—just don't try to walk backward, or you'll land smack on your behind.

If you hit a patch of ice and slide or lose your balance, fall gently onto your side to avoid a tumble. It's the same "bail-out" fall you use when cross-country skiing, snowboarding, or surfing, taking advantage of the soft, wide surface of your flank to break your fall. You'll land in a crouched position on the snow. From here, you can use your arms and poles to push yourself until your weight is over your boots and stand upright.

After tromping through the snow for a quarter of an hour, your body will cry out for a break. That's okay: the cold, exertion, and altitude really work your body, especially during pregnancy. Rest and hydrate. Slow your pace by taking smaller steps if you begin to feel short of breath. Make enjoying the scenery your goal as much as getting to the end of the trail, so you relish the slow pace and pauses rather than becoming frustrated.

Cooling Down

When you reach the end of the trail, panting and jubilant, take a few minutes to cool down before flopping down in the car with some snacks and cranking up the heat. Slowly bring your heart rate down to resting and gently stretch the muscles you have been using so they don't get tight and sore later. Five to ten minutes of walking with easy steps in your boots or snowshoes on packed snow (while you chug a bottle of water) will cool you down. Good hydration will also help flush out the lactic acid that has built up in those tired muscles, causing soreness. Then, try some stretches, focusing on limbering up your legs, hips, arms, and back. Snowshoeing increases the blood flow to your legs, so you may find that your ankles swell up a bit afterward. Just take off your shoes and socks when you get home and put your feet up on the sofa or a chair to help get that extra fluid pumped back to your heart.

Equipment Considerations

Snowshoeing requires no ultra-cool clothing, no gear hype, no specialized boots (waterproof hiking boots are best) or poles (alpine, cross-country, backcountry, or no poles at all will work), and little hassle. You don't even need a lift ticket to take advantage of stunning trails and breathtaking vistas. All you need is some snowshoes—and rentals will do just fine.

My only strong recommendation for choosing snowshoes is to go with something modern; old-fashioned wooden and leather snowshoes, though romantic, are giant and cumbersome and will wear you out in minutes. Modern snowshoes are light, sleek, shaped to allow you to walk normally, and easy to use. Choosing a snowshoe really depends on the conditions you're heading into—powder requires a shoe with more "float." During pregnancy, you've gained some weight, which may also affect your choice of snowshoe: the heavier you are (or more weight you are carrying), the more float you need so you don't sink deeply into the snow.

If you have a choice, choose a narrower or tapered snowshoe because it is easier to walk in and allows you to have a more natural gait. The rounder snowshoes float better on powder but force your legs farther apart, putting more strain on your hips. This can get uncomfortable during pregnancy, when those joints are relaxed and the muscles supporting them can get strained. If you're walking on well-packed snow, you can try asymmetrical snowshoes, which are even easier on your hips because they allow you to keep your feet closer together.

As with all winter outdoor activities, dress in peelable layers. Your underwear is just as important as your jacket, and moisture wicking counts for a whole lot more than fashion sense. Cotton undies and t-shirts will first get soaked with sweat and then get cold. Synthetic fabrics, like polypropylene, are best for keeping you warm and dry. Some women prefer fleece bras and spandex cycling shorts to prevent chafing.

Because, you're going to heat up and then cool down drastically when you take a break or get out in the wind, make sure the next layer can come off and fit in your pack or tie around your waist easily; a fleece or wool layer is a good idea. Your jacket should repel water and stop wind. And pay special attention to your hands and feet, since they are most susceptible to cold, blisters, and getting wet; wear thermal socks and mittens and waterproof boots and gloves. Don't head out without a warm hat, neck gaiter or scarf, gloves, and some UV-protective sunglasses, a supply of extra lip balm, and a generous layer of SPF-30 sweat-proof sunscreen.

Preparing for Difficult Situations

The main advantage of traveling well-established and frequented trails is avoiding winter hazards. Trails that were peaceful and clearly visible in the summer may be fraught with hazards in the snow, like hidden ditches, fallen logs, fast-moving streams, and snow-laden trees. The trail itself may be nearly impossible to locate without familiar landmarks or a worn path. Crossing frozen streams and lakes or traversing avalanche country is simply dangerous. Be careful not to step in water—several pounds of powder can freeze onto a wet shoe. And avoid snowshoeing in steep areas after a snowstorm, which is when the majority of avalanches occur, or in warmer weather, which often precipitates avalanches. Even a small avalanche is very dangerous—a layer only six inches deep and twenty feet wide can slide downhill a hundred feet and bury a person.

Snowshoeing trails in parks and resorts are marked with signs or flags well above the snowline. If it's groomed or has been recently used by other snowshoers or cross-country skiers, you can easily follow the others' packed prints to stay on track, keep up speed, and save energy. Although snowmobile paths are also good routes, make sure you have room to get out of the way quickly in case a vehicle comes along.

Check the weather before you head out; storms often hit in the afternoon and dense fog or blowing snow can make it impossible for you to find your trail. Find out the highest elevation on the trail—it should be below eight thousand feet, and you should have already spent a few days getting used to the altitude before exerting yourself on the trail.

snowshoeing

Planning Pointers for Pregnancy

1 Take your time. You can learn to snowshoe during pregnancy, but it takes some conditioning. The basic skills are no different from walking, but the workout is much more intense. If you haven't been doing a lot of aerobic exercise this pregnancy, go slowly and take breaks to catch your breath. The stronger you feel, the safer you'll be on the trail.

2 Snowshoe a familiar trail. Make sure you have a map, recognize regular markers, and follow another person's footsteps. Pay attention to prominent landmarks on the way. Wandering off trail or trying to locate a trail hidden under snow is difficult and risky because of unexpected winter hazards. Remember, it gets dark much sooner, you can't move very fast, and the temperature can plummet quickly.

3 Conserve energy. Let someone more energetic break the path and tromp down the powder in front of you. Stick to packed trails or step directly in the footsteps of the leader. If you begin to feel tired, take smaller steps and take breaks. Consuming nutritious snacks and lots of water will also help keep your energy up.

4 Fall safely. Since you set your own pace when snowshoeing for fun, you are not likely to fall. You may even want to take poles along for extra balance. But if you do hit a slippery patch or lose your balance, bend your knees and try to fall onto your side (ideally into a forgiving snow bank), where the impact of the fall is distributed on your flank and you are less likely to hurt yourself.

5 Train on your off days. Let snowshoeing motivate you to stay in great shape during pregnancy. If you can't make it to a snowshoeing trail this week or if the snow's too slushy, try hiking instead.

6 Focus on posture. Keeping good posture when snowshoeing helps build your everyday posture and prevents back pain down the road.

7 Pick easily removable layers that wick away moisture. Warm, dry underwear is as important as a water- and windproof outer shell. Stay away from cotton and bulky layers that are hard to take off. Make sure your head, neck, feet, and hands are well protected.

8 Prevent the burn. That reflective snow, altitude, wind, and sun can really damage your sensitive skin. Use plenty of SPF-30 sweat-proof sunscreen and lip balm. And wear goggles or UV-protective sunglasses for the glare.

9 Banish your winter blues. Fresh air, spectacular scenery, meditative silence, and some good company are an amazing salve for grouchy moods and low spirits. Exploring a pristine landscape on snowshoes can be as easy as stepping out your front door or getting to the local park. Snowshoeing is also a more relaxing and safer alternative to skiing. The exercise does wonders for your attitude and is about as good as it gets for your pregnancy, too. If you decide to make snow-shoeing a regular part of your winter workout, you'll be in prime shape for delivery—and eager to bring your baby when you return to the wilderness.

POSTPARTUM WEIGHT
CHANGES

• • •

EXCERCISE AND
BREASTFEEDING

• • •

RESUMING ACTIVITY
AFTER DELIVERY

• • •

POSTPARTUM TONING
EXCERCISES

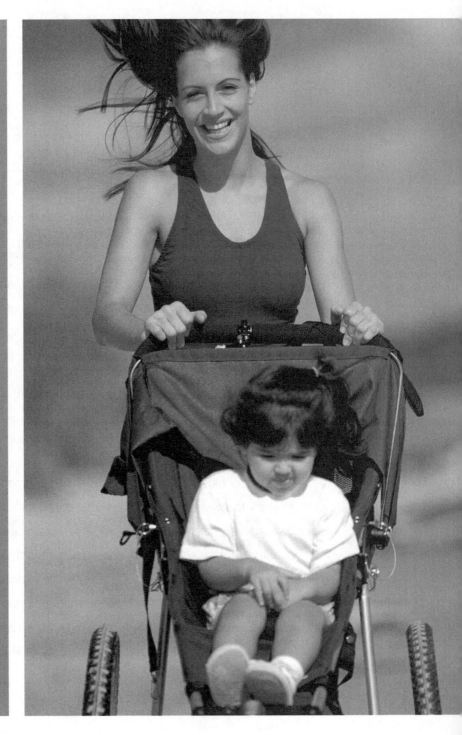

Recovering and Resuming Activity

Starting up an exercise regimen after delivery—whether it is days or weeks later—is a healthy way to get some time out of the house and get in touch with yourself. But taking care of a newborn is hard work and you may find yourself feeling too worn out to begin exercise in the weeks right after delivery. Give yourself time.

Your body recovers slowly from delivery, especially if you had a cesarean birth or any complications around the birth. Your body itself takes four to six weeks to get back to its pre-pregnancy physiology. Weight gain and deconditioning make resuming exercise challenging. The effects of relaxin, the hormone that causes joint and ligament laxity during pregnancy, can persist for up to three months after delivery, contributing to your risk of injuries such as a sprained ankle. Although you can safely start gentle exercise, like stretching and walking, within a day or two after giving birth, getting back into a regular exercise schedule can take months.

Being responsible for a newborn affects your eating habits, your sleep schedule, and your ability to allocate time for anything else. Even committed athletes find it difficult to resume the level of activity they enjoyed during pregnancy. But the postpartum period also supplies a rare opportunity to reestablish healthy lifestyle habits. Think about it: you are restructuring every aspect of your life anyway. Plus, you may be particularly motivated by the desire to return to your previous size and shape, to boost your energy level, and to reduce stress.

If you did stay active during pregnancy, you have a head start and will probably get back in shape more quickly. Most women who were active during pregnancy continue to exercise after their babies are born. And 70 percent of these women are actually in better shape a year after delivery than they were before pregnancy! A study of German champion women athletes showed that most made objective improvements in performance after pregnancy and childbirth. Andrea Mead Lawrence, the famed American alpine skier, captured two Gold medals at the winter Olympics, had three children in the next four years, and qualified for the next Olympics a mere four months after her son was born. She finished in a tie for fourth place in the giant slalom, a tenth of a second behind the Bronze winner.

Fitness is only one of the many ways you benefit from postpartum exercise. Staying active after delivery will also help you to have better bladder control, build stronger bones, prevent constipation, and improve your mood. Depression is common after delivery and can be devastating. Regular exercise may help your body deal better with the rapidly changing hormone levels and resulting mood swings.

Many women join "mommy groups" where they can exercise with their babies and share the experience with other new mothers. Look for swimming (newborns are surprisingly happy in the water) and walking groups that involve your baby or offer child care. Trade baby-sitting favors so you can get out without your baby too. Even a short hike or bike ride can really clear your mind and reenergize you. For many active women, getting out to do the activities they love is part of being a good parent and setting a good example. But remember to do it for yourself as well: this is your time.

Postpartum Weight Changes

On average, women maintain a couple of pounds (about 1 kg) of extra weight after delivery. That's not much, but over 70 percent of women feel unhappy about their physical shape six months after giving birth. A few factors contribute to the likelihood of retaining weight after delivery. According to an article in the *American Journal of Public Health*, women who have had more than one child or who are over age thirty-five are more likely to retain postpartum weight. Women who take a longer maternity leave tend to lose less weight than women who return to work sooner. Also, women who gain excessive weight during pregnancy are more likely to keep some of that extra weight after delivery.

But regardless of the women's age, race, pre-pregnancy weight, number of previous pregnancies, or pregnancy weight gain, one factor plays a significant role in predicting postpartum fitness: exercise. As the journal *Clinics in Sports Medicine* reports, 30 percent more of active women (compared to nonexercising women) return to their pre-pregnancy weight within a year of delivery. And even more of these women return to their original fat levels and abdominal tone.

Although you may have heard that losing pregnancy pounds takes nine months—corresponding to the nine months that it took to gain them—you will probably lose that weight much faster. In fact, you lose most of your pregnancy weight in the first three months after delivery. Simply delivering your baby and the placenta causes a loss of about ten to thirteen pounds (4.5 to 5.8 kg). In the week after delivery, sweating, shedding lochia (the remainder of the endometrial lining inside your uterus), and shrinking of the uterus causes another seven to eleven pounds (3.2 to 5.0 kg) of weight loss. Returning to your previous activity level in the few months after having your baby takes care of most of the rest. Between three and six months after delivery, average weight loss is only about 2.2 pounds (1 kg).

A combination of a healthy diet and a regular exercise routine is the best way to recover your fitness level, according to an article in the *American Journal of Clinical Nutrition*. After your baby is born, your body naturally readjusts to its new caloric needs—meaning you'll eat a bit less since you don't need all those calories to maintain the pregnancy. Keep in mind that you'll still need to eat more than before pregnancy if you are breastfeeding. As long as you don't overeat and you stay moderately active, you'll steadily lose weight.

Exercise and Breastfeeding

Many women continue to breastfeed for months and even years after delivery—while they are also getting back to work and getting back in shape. In fact, breastfeeding is an important part of recovering after delivery, since it helps your uterus contract and return to its original size (that's why you may feel cramping when you breastfeed, especially in the first few weeks). Breastfeeding also uses a lot of calories.

Breast milk is very healthy for your baby. Don't pass up this unique opportunity to bond with your child and pass on some good immune protection. A regular moderate workout should not interfere with your breastfeeding schedule and may help you sleep better between feedings. Even world-class athletes have competed in international competitions within three months of delivering while breastfeeding everyday.

If you are eager to resume exercise, you can do so safely while breastfeeding if you take a few precautions. Make time to sleep enough, eat sufficient amounts, and drink a lot of water. You may notice that you have sore nipples or a somewhat reduced milk supply initially—but that is easily preventable.

Some women find that they produce less milk if they exercise regularly. Surprisingly, this is not because they are burning so many calories that they don't have enough to pass on to the baby. Studies reported in the journal *Seminars in Perinatology* show that regular exercise and maternal weight loss of about a pound per week from weeks four to fourteen after delivery have no effect on the breastfed infant's growth. The decrease in a woman's milk supply is also not because a tight sports bra constricts the breasts. Instead, exercise can cause a reduction in a mother's milk supply because of dehydration. You may produce less milk after exercising simply because you are too dry.

Keep in mind that you are drinking for two: you need to take in all the fluids your body *and* your baby need. When you exercise while breastfeeding, you need more fluids than you did during pregnancy and certainly a lot more than before pregnancy. Keep a bottle of water handy and drink at least a liter of water per hour while you are exercising and even more in hot or humid weather. Staying well hydrated will help you to give your baby a healthy supply of breast milk.

Unless your doctor specifically recommends it, don't supplement your baby's feedings with formula just because you are exercising and concerned that he may not be getting enough milk. In fact, adding formula will just cause your body to produce less milk overall, because most babies will choose a bottle over the breast since it gives more milk with less effort. And the less your baby nurses, the less milk your body makes.

If you find that your baby is not as eager to breastfeed right after you exercise, it could be the lactic acid in your milk. If you enjoyed a long, hard workout, then your muscles were producing lactic acid, a by-product of their activity. The lactic acid shows up in your breast milk (for up to ninety minutes after a strenuous workout) and your baby may not like its taste. If your baby drinks it right up, don't worry, lactic acid won't have any harmful effects.

Your breasts, when full of milk, may be sore when you exercise. Toward the end of pregnancy, your breast tissue becomes fully developed and your breasts may weigh a pound or more—each! A couple of days after delivery, your breasts fill with milk and become even larger and more cumbersome. Over the next few months your breasts do get smaller, as they (and your baby) become more efficient at the whole breastfeeding process. Exercising with those heavy breasts in those first few weeks can be uncomfortable, especially if you haven't breastfed for a couple of hours. For this reason, try breastfeeding before exercising.

You may also find that your nipples rub against the bra and become tender. Make sure you are wearing a well-fitting nursing bra—those maternity bras just won't be comfortable anymore. Also, try wearing soft nursing pads over your nipples to protect them from chafing. Some athletes also recommend rubbing your nipples with petroleum jelly (or lanolin or colostrum cream) before heading out—this is especially helpful if your nipples are dry and cracked.

As soon as you feel up to it, get out there and gradually resume some of your favorite activities. Even if you're breastfeeding, you don't want to abandon the good habits you developed during pregnancy or lose this opportunity to get back in shape. Both breastfeeding and exercise are important parts of your recovery—and of getting your motherhood started on the healthiest track.

Resuming Activity After Delivery

As your body slowly recovers from delivery, you'll feel like doing something active to start getting back in shape and get out of the house. Talk with your doctor before you start up an exercise regimen after delivery to make sure you don't have to watch out for anything special. For example, if you had a cesarean delivery, a deep vaginal tear, or unusual bleeding after delivery, your doctor may ask you to rest for a few weeks before exerting yourself. On average, women start getting active again about two weeks after delivery—but it varies from three days to eight weeks. I recommend starting gentle activity a few days after delivery and establishing a regular exercise routine about two weeks later. Don't try to resume your pre-pregnancy (or even pregnancy) workout right away: ramp up gradually. Remember that the time you took for delivery and recovery has deconditioned you a bit, so take it easy.

In the day or two after delivery, take advantage of your stay in the hospital to get some rest. This doesn't mean you should stay in bed for two days straight, however. While you are in the hospital, your obstetrician will encourage you to walk if you can. Even though your vaginal or abdominal area may feel tender, walking will not cause cesarean or episiotomy stitches to come loose. Just walking the halls (to and from the nursery, for example) helps your body recover from the delivery and stretches your tired muscles. And walking helps prevent constipation, heartburn, and infection immediately after delivery. In the first week after a vaginal or C-section delivery, try doing some toning exercises, described below, to activate your major muscle groups and tone those sore, stretched-out pelvic muscles.

For most women, the most comfortable way to ease back into exercise after delivery is to start walking. Once you get home, starting a couple of days after delivery, try walking around the neighborhood at least three times per week for fifteen to twenty minutes at a time. Walking is especially healthy because it is a weight-bearing and an aerobic exercise; it is gentle on your joints, pelvis, and heart; and you can bring your baby with you, in a stroller, sling, or front pack.

At about two weeks after a vaginal delivery or four weeks after a c-section, if you feel ready, you can ramp up your exercise routine—choose activities that get your heart rate up but that don't feel strenuous like longer walks, hikes, biking, or kayaking. If you had any stitches or staples (after a cesarean or an episiotomy), make sure they are removed or healed (most vaginal sutures are absorbed by your body) before you do any water activities so that you avoid infection. Also avoid any abdominal exercises while you have cesarean stitches or staples in place. Aim for a half-hour workout at least four times a week. In the month or two after delivery, try swimming, snowshoeing, or running. And if you feel like in-line skating or cross-country skiing, go for it! Just listen to your body and limit your excursions to an hour at a time, with regular breaks for hydration and cooling down.

By six to eight weeks after delivery, if you feel ready, you can get back to the strenuous activities you avoided during pregnancy, like training, racing, sprinting, and just pushing yourself hard again. Now that your body has recovered fully, you may notice that you have more stamina than you did before pregnancy. Many athletes find that they are able to achieve a higher level of fitness after accomplishing that marathon of pregnancy and delivery.

Postpartum Toning Exercises

Pregnancy and delivery are tough on your body. Your back is exhausted, your abdomen looks nothing like it did before pregnancy, and you ache in places you never paid attention to before. Muscles that you didn't know existed, like those pelvic muscles that you use to hold in your urine, are tender, stretched, and not working right (incontinence is common after delivery). The few weeks after you leave the hospital are the perfect time to focus on toning these muscles. You can get started with the exercises below as soon as you get home.

A regular, gentle postpartum toning routine takes about fifteen minutes a day. You can use hand weights (try five-, eight-, or ten-pound free weights in each hand) or even hold your baby, if you feel comfortable, when doing some of these exercises. All you need is a little floor space, ideally with carpet or an exercise mat.

Pelvic Toning

Kegel Exercises: Whatever exercises you do after delivery, throw in a few Kegel exercises to help strengthen your pelvic floor muscles. Kegels tighten the muscles that you used to support the uterus and to push out the baby if you had a vaginal delivery. Most women experience some incontinence (leaking urine) after delivery and half of all women experience some incontinence later in life—Kegels help prevent this problem.

You can do Kegels anytime—whether you are standing, sitting, or lying down—and no one will know you are doing them (although your partner may enjoy your doing Kegels during lovemaking since tightening those muscles increases vaginal pressure on the penis).

Squeeze the muscles around your vagina and anus as if you are holding in urine. Hold it in for a second, release, and repeat. At first, holding for a second or two is challenging, but as the muscles grow stronger you'll be able to control the movement better. Do ten Kegels in a row, holding each for a couple seconds before relaxing and repeating.

Pelvic Bridge: Lie on your back with your knees bent and your feet flat on the ground. Your arms should lie alongside your body. Pull in your abdominal muscles, squeeze your buttocks, and lift your hips up toward the ceiling until your buttocks and entire back are off the ground. In this position, supported only by your feet and shoulders (forming a bridge or, more accurately, a ramp), squeeze and release your buttocks, pulsing your pelvis toward the ceiling. Repeat, pulsing ten times. Then release your body back onto the ground and repeat the whole sequence. Do three sets of ten pulsations.

Arm and Chest Toning

Chest Presses: Lying on your back, with your legs bent and your feet on the floor, hold your weights, or your baby, straight up in front of you and gently lower down with your elbows pointing out to the sides. Then push up and repeat ten times. Complete three sets of ten chest presses.

Bicep Curls: Stand with your back straight, your abdominals pulled in, your pelvis tucked under you, and your feet about shoulder-width apart. Holding a weight in each hand, or holding your baby around her chest below her underarms, keep your elbows anchored at your waist and curl your forearms up toward your chest. Then relax until your elbows are at right angles again. Repeat ten times. Complete three sets of ten curls.

Abdominal Toning

Abdominal Crunches: Lie on your back (with your baby sitting on your stomach and supported by your thighs, if you wish) with your knees bent. Contract your abdominals and lift your shoulders and head off the ground. Rather than using your neck to pull your shoulders off the ground (since touching your chin to your chest during curls will strain your neck), keep your spine and neck in line and contract your belly to lift your upper body. Hold for five seconds, then release your head and shoulders back to the ground. Repeat ten times. Complete two sets of ten crunches. As your build these abdominal muscles, increase the number of sets to five, for a total of fifty crunches.

Abdominal Curls: Lie on your back with your hips and knees both bent at right angles. Your thighs should be perpendicular to the floor and your calves should be parallel to the floor, with your feet off the ground. Curl your head and shoulders toward your knees. Use your abdominals to keep your legs at right angles as you lift your shoulders off the ground. When your shoulders are off the ground, your abdominal muscles should be firm; hold this position for five seconds. Release and repeat ten times. Complete two sets of ten repetitions.

Once your abdominal muscles are stronger, you can extend your legs so that you are in a V-shape, with your legs straight, your feet a foot or two off the ground, and your chest and head elevated. Instead of curling, just hold this position for fifteen seconds. Repeat three times.

Plank Position: Lie on your belly, then flex your toes so that your toe pads are on the floor and bend your elbows alongside your body with your hands next to your face. Push your torso, hips, and legs into a plank position so that only your toes and forearms are on the floor, keeping your back flat. You can clasp your fingers together on the floor for improved balance. Tighten your abdominals and your buttocks. Hold this position for fifteen seconds. Repeat three times.

Leg Toning

Squats: Stand with your feet shoulder-width apart. Holding weights in your hands straight out to your sides or holding your baby close to your chest, squat down as if you are sitting in an invisible chair. Keep your knees above your toes and your back straight. Hold for three seconds. Then straighten to standing. Repeat ten times. If you do these exercises regularly, you should be able to gradually increase the number of sets you do until you can do three sets of ten squats with a brief break between sets.

Pliés: Stand with your legs about three feet apart, with your toes and knees aimed outward. Bend your legs so that you are tightening your thighs and so that each knee goes over the corresponding foot. Keep your back straight and your pelvis tucked under you. Hold for ten seconds. Then, gently lift just the heel of one foot and squat deeper. Hold for another ten. Put that heel down, stand, and repeat, lifting the other heel this time. Repeat ten times. For added resistance, hold weights straight out to your sides or hold your baby to your chest.

Leg Lifts: Sitting on a bench or chair, lift one leg up so that it is extended straight out in front of you. Gently raise the leg a few inches, so that your thigh comes off the chair and your knee remains straight. You'll feel your thigh, buttock, and abdominal muscles tighten as you lift. Relax, and repeat ten times on one side, then ten on the other. Complete two sets of ten on each side. If you hold your baby on the thigh you are working, do two sets of five lifts on each side and complete two sets.

Even though you may feel impossibly busy and exhausted, sneak in at least a few minutes for these simple toning exercises—they'll take less time than one of your newborn's frequent naps. Toning will help your body recover from delivery and will help you pay attention to your own body.

When you feel up to it, exercise after delivery to improve your fitness, relieve stress, tone your body, and just to get away from it all. Have fun. Bring friends along. Go somewhere beautiful, even if it's the park around the corner. Your exercise time can be a fun and educational experience for your baby, too. Part of parenting is sharing your active lifestyle and your passion for nature. The outdoors is a rich classroom for a child; take time to appreciate and show your child the small, fascinating aspects of nature along the way, like the feel of cool water or the movement of a trail of ants. Plus, involving your child in your healthy habits will encourage her to play outside and view exercise as an essential—and enjoyable—part of the day, just as you do.

Glossary

Abruption: The premature detachment of the placenta from the uterine wall. Abruption can occur for many reasons, including trauma, a defect in the placenta, and cocaine use.

Aerobic exercise: Exercise that conditions the heart and lungs. This type of exercise uses aerobic metabolism, meaning your muscles depend on oxygen to function, therefore conditioning your heart and lungs, too. Examples of aerobic exercise are swimming, jogging, and cross-country skiing.

Anaerobic exercise: Exercise that is so strenuous that your muscles do not have enough oxygen to function, causing buildup of lactic acid and severe fatigue and endangering the blood flow to the fetus. Examples of anaerobic exercise include sprinting, racing, and exercising to the point of complete exhaustion.

Anemia: A condition in which the number of red blood cells or oxygen-carrying materials in blood is low, causing shortness of breath, pale skin, and fatigue. The most common cause of anemia in adults is low iron levels.

Apgar score: A system of evaluating a newborn's physical health by assigning a value to five criteria: heart rate, respiratory effort, muscle tone, response to stimuli, and color.

Bag of water: The amnionic (or amniotic) sac that surrounds the fetus and contains the amniotic fluid. When the bag of water breaks, the amniotic fluid leaks out through the vagina, indicating that labor is in progress.

Bloody show: The passage of thick, blood-tinged mucus that often precedes the onset of cervical dilation with labor. Near the due date, seeing this bloody show means that labor will start soon.

Blood sugar: The level of carbohydrates, including glucose, galactose, and lactose, in the bloodstream. These sugars provide short-term energy for the body.

Bradycardia: Slowness of the heartbeat. Although the fetus's heartbeat constantly fluctuates, a consistently low heart rate can signify a problem. A very fit adult may have a low heart rate because her heart is well conditioned; in this case, the relatively slow heart rate is healthy.

Braxton Hicks contractions: Rhythmic activity of the uterine muscle that does not lead to labor. These contractions are brief, do not increase in intensity or frequency, and typically resolve after a few minutes with rest.

Breaking the bag of water: Rupture of the amniotic membranes, or the bag of water, that releases the amniotic fluid, causing a gush or a trickle of fluid from the vagina and signifying the onset of labor.

Carbohydrate: An organic food substance that includes starches, sugars, and cellulose. Common sources of carbohydrates are grains, fruits, vegetables, and sugars. Carbohydrates are broken down into glucose, a sugar that provides energy for the body.

Cesarean section: Operative delivery of the baby through an incision in the abdominal wall and uterus. Also called a C-section, or abdominal delivery.

Contractions: Rhythmic activity of the uterine muscle that eventually causes the dilation of the cervix and delivery of the baby. Contractions can be felt as a tightening across the abdomen or cramping in the pelvis or lower back, or, very early in labor, not felt at all but detectable with a contraction monitor (tocometer).

Cryptosporidium: A microscopic protozoan that lives in the intestines of animals, including farm animals, that can cause an infection in humans. This infection is most common in people who have contact with farm animals, such as cattle, but can be contracted from contact with contaminated dirt. The infection causes diarrhea, fever, and abdominal pain.

Deep vein thrombosis (DVT): A blood clot in a large vein, typically in the leg or arm. The clot causes blockage of the blood vessel, resulting in pain, numbness, and swelling.

Dextrose: A form of sugar or glucose found in plants and animals and which is a breakdown product of starches.

Diabetes: Diabetes mellitus is a disorder of sugar metabolism in which the body is unable to regulate sugar levels because of inadequate or ineffective insulin (the hormone that controls sugar levels). Untreated diabetes in pregnancy can have significant effects on the developing fetus, including birth defects.

Diastasis recti: Separation of the muscles of the abdominal wall (the rectus muscles). Diastasis recti can occur during pregnancy because of strain to the abdominal muscles.

Dynamic stretches: Smooth movements that improve the flexibility of your muscles and prepare you for exercise by increasing blood flow to specific muscle groups.

Ectopic pregnancy: A pregnancy located outside the uterus. The most common location is in the fallopian tubes, where the growing fetus can rupture the tube, causing internal bleeding and requiring emergency surgery.

Edema: Fluid collection in the soft tissues, causing swelling. During pregnancy, fluid moves into the subcutaneous tissue under the skin, causing gradual swelling in the ankles and even in the hands and arms. Edema that develops suddenly may indicate a problem, such as preeclampsia.

Electrolytes: Trace mineral substances, including as sodium, potassium, and calcium, that are necessary for normal body function. Sweating, inadequate nutrition, and illnesses such as diabetes can affect your levels of electrolytes.

Endorphins: Hormones that stimulate opioid receptors in the brain (acting like narcotics similar to morphine) and affect pain perception, mood, and energy level.

Episiotomy: An incision of the vagina and surrounding tissue during vaginal delivery to create room for the fetal head and to prevent traumatic and irregular tearing of the vagina.

Fallopian tube: The tube connecting the ovary to the uterus. The egg travels from the ovary down the fallopian tube. Fertilization most commonly occurs in the fallopian tubes and the fertilized egg then travels to the uterus, where it implants and continues to develop.

False labor contraction: Contraction of the uterine muscle that does not result in labor or dilation of the cervix. False labor can be distinguished from true labor because the contractions do not become stronger or more regular and typically resolve with rest. False labor contractions are also known as Braxton Hicks contractions.

Fetal growth restriction: Lower-than-expected measurement of the fetus based on standardized fetal weight and gestational age tables. The fetus's weight can be estimated roughly by measuring the uterine size (a tape measure from the pubic bone to the top of the uterus can be used to help track fetal growth) and can be determined more accurately with ultrasound measurements. Many factors can contribute to low fetal growth measurements, including maternal illness, drug or alcohol abuse, poor nutrition, fetal infection, multiple pregnancy (twins), and inaccurate fetal dating.

Fetal stress: Fetal distress caused by factors such as infection, placental bleeding, or a difficult or prolonged labor. Signs of fetal stress, such as low heart rate, meconium-stained amniotic fluid early in labor, or decreased fetal movement, may indicate a need for a more urgent delivery.

Forceps delivery: Vaginal delivery using metal forceps, instruments shaped somewhat like salad tongs, to help deliver the fetal head.

Frostbite: Damage to the skin and tissue below the skin from exposure to low temperatures. Frostbite results in loss of sensation and blood flow and can result in permanent injury.

Frostnip: Damage to the superficial layer of the skin from exposure to low temperatures, resulting in redness, temporary sensation loss, and blistering.

Gestational diabetes: Disorder of sugar metabolism occurring only during pregnancy because of changes in the body's ability to store sugar. Uncontrolled gestational diabetes can result in abnormally high blood sugar, which can affect fetal development.

Giardia lamblia: A species of protozoan commonly found in untreated fresh water, such as mountain streams, which can cause intestinal infection. Common symptoms include diarrhea and abdominal cramping.

Glucose: A natural sugar found in fruits and milk, that is the chief source of energy for the body. Extra glucose is stored in muscles and fat and released to the bloodstream when the body needs more energy. Glucose is also known as dextrose or blood sugar.

Heat exhaustion: An effect of excessive exposure to heat, resulting in dizziness, low body temperature, headache, nausea, and even collapse.

Heat stroke: A condition that develops from excess heat exposure resulting in dangerously high body temperature, muscle cramps, dizziness, headache, and dry skin.

Hematocrit: A measurement of the number of red blood cells in the blood. A low hematocrit indicates anemia.

Hyperglycemia: High blood sugar level. Blood sugar can rise temporarily after a large meal, but a consistently elevated blood sugar may indicate difficulty storing sugar, such as with diabetes.

Hyperthermia: High body temperature. This can result from excess heat exposure or physical exertion. If the body produces heat faster than it can release it, the body's core temperature can rise, dangerously affecting the fetus.

Hypoglycemia: Low blood sugar level. Low sugar can result from missing meals or inadequate snacking, especially with the increased calorie requirements of pregnancy. Low sugar can also occur with exercise, when the body uses up blood sugar to power the muscles.

Hypothermia: Low body temperature. Exposure to cold, windy, and wet conditions can result in low body temperature.

Incompetent cervix: A condition in which the cervix starts to dilate prematurely (before the fetus is viable) during pregnancy, often resulting in miscarriage. In a patient with a known history of cervical incompetence, a cerclage, or stitch around the cervix, can be placed to prevent the cervix from opening early.

Incontinence: Inability to control urine or stool function. Urinary incontinence is common during and after pregnancy because the muscles around the bladder are stretched.

Insulin: A hormone produced by the pancreas that helps the body regulate sugar levels. When blood sugar levels are high, insulin is released to tell the body to store the extra sugar in muscles and fat to be used later. In a person with diabetes, insulin levels are low or ineffective, so sugar levels stay abnormally high.

Kegel exercises: Exercises performed to strengthen the pelvic muscles. To do Kegels, repeatedly contract and release your pelvic muscles as if you are trying to stop yourself from urinating. Kegel exercises help improve vaginal tone after a vaginal delivery and help prevent and treat urinary incontinence.

Kick count: A method of measuring fetal well-being by counting the number of fetal movements over a period of time. Typically, a fetus should move at least four times in an hour. Movements should be measured while the mother is lying comfortably on her left side and focusing on fetal activity.

Lactic acid: A product of anaerobic metabolism during strenuous muscle exertion. Heavy muscle use breaks down a sugar called glycogen and releases lactic acid. Buildup of lactic acid in muscles causes muscle cramping. In diabetics, skipping meals or missing insulin doses can result in very high acid levels (ketoacidosis) because of the breakdown of muscles for energy.

Linea alba: The slightly pale line running vertically between the belly button and the pubic bone. It is the line where the two abdominal muscles (the rectus muscles) come together.

Lochia: Vaginal discharge of blood, mucus, and tissue following childbirth.

Lordosis: A curvature of the spine resulting in a forward curve, or arch, of the lower back. This posture is common in pregnancy, when the weight of the belly pulls the lower part of the spine forward.

Mastitis: Inflammation of the breast or the mammary (milk-producing) tissue.

Meconium: An infant's first intestinal discharge. It is black-green and consists of mucus and bile. Passage of meconium typically occurs after birth but can precede delivery, resulting a green-tinged and soupy amniotic fluid.

Melasma: Patchy discoloration of the skin which can occur during pregnancy due to hormonal changes.

Miscarriage: Loss of a pregnancy before the fetus is viable (before about twenty-four weeks). This is also called a spontaneous abortion.

Nonstress test (NST): A measurement of fetal well-being. A monitor on the mother's abdomen records the fetal heart rate in response to fetal movement. With movement, the fetus's heart rate should increase temporarily. A normal, or "reactive," nonstress test shows at least two elevations in fetal heart rate within a twenty-minute period.

Normal spontaneous vaginal delivery: Delivery of an infant vaginally without the use of forceps or vacuum devices.

Oral rehydration solution: A mixture of water, salt, and sugar that helps replenish electrolytes and prevent dehydration. Store-bought rehydration drinks, such as sports drinks, also contain other electrolytes than one can lose with sweating, such as potassium.

Ovary: The female organ that stores and releases eggs and produces the female hormones, including estrogen and progesterone. One walnut-sized ovary is located on each side of the pelvis and each is connected to the uterus by a fallopian tube.

Oxytocin: A natural hormone, released by the brain during labor, that helps stimulate uterine contractions to be stronger and more regular. Oxytocin also stimulates breast milk release. A synthetic oxytocin (Pitocin) can be given intravenously or intramuscularly to help stimulate labor, increase the force of contractions, or help the uterus to contract and control bleeding after delivery.

Pitocin: A synthetic (or animal-derived) hormone that acts like oxytocin and can be given to stimulate labor, increase the force and regularity of contractions during labor, or help the uterus to contract after delivery to prevent bleeding.

Placenta: The organ joining the mother and fetus and allowing exchange of nutrients, oxygen, and waste products. The fetus is attached to the placenta by the umbilical cord and the placenta is attached to the mother's uterus. At term, the placenta is about sixteen centimeters across and two centimeters thick.

Placenta previa: A placenta that develops in the lower part of the uterus, over the cervical opening. With a previa late in pregnancy, any dilation or disturbance of the cervix can cause placental bleeding.

Placental abruption: The premature detachment of the placenta from the uterine wall. Placental abruption can occur for many reasons, including trauma, a defect in the placenta, and cocaine use.

Potable: Fit to drink. In a campground or park, water labeled "potable" has been treated (like city water) for safety.

Preeclampsia: A complication of pregnancy that causes swelling (or edema), high blood pressure, and protein in the urine. Delivery of the fetus resolves preeclampsia.

Pregnancy-induced hypertension (PIH): Elevated blood pressure occurring only during pregnancy. If untreated, high blood pressure can affect the health of the placenta and fetal growth.

Premature delivery: Delivery of an infant between twenty and thirty-six weeks of gestation.

Preterm labor: Signs of labor (cramps, backache, pelvic pressure, rupture of membranes), contractions, and cervical dilation before thirty-six weeks of gestation.

Pyelonephritis: A kidney infection that typically develops from a bacterial infection in the urinary tract and bladder. Urinary tract infections are more common during pregnancy because sugar in the urine helps bacteria grow.

Relaxin: A hormone secreted during pregnancy that helps to relax ligaments and soften the cervix for childbirth.

Rupture of membranes: Tear of the amniotic membranes that releases the amniotic fluid, causing a gush or a trickle of fluid from the vagina and signifying the onset of labor. This is also known as breaking the bag of water.

Spontaneous Abortion: Natural loss of a pregnancy before about twenty-four weeks. Also called miscarriage.

Spotting: Small amount of vaginal bleeding. During pregnancy, spotting can be caused by many things, including infection, trauma to the cervix, disruption of the placenta, or the onset of labor.

Sprain: An injury to a ligament (the tissue that connects bones) caused by abnormal or excessive force to a joint.

Strain: An injury to a muscle caused by overuse or improper use.

Term: Between thirty-seven and forty-two weeks of gestation (calculated from the first day of the last period). The due date is the first day of the fortieth week of gestation.

Tidal volume: The amount of air that is inspired (breathed in) or expired (breathed out) in a single breath during regular breathing.

Tubal pregnancy: A pregnancy located in the fallopian tube, not in the uterus. A fetus will not be able to develop or survive in the fallopian tube and it can cause maternal pain and internal bleeding, requiring emergency surgery.

Uterus: The female muscular organ in which the fertilized egg implants and the fetus develops and grows. The uterus supplies the placenta with blood flow and nutrients to support the fetus. During labor, the muscular walls of the uterus rhythmically contract, pushing the fetus out through the vagina.

Weight-bearing exercise: Activity in which the majority of your weight is supported by your legs, such as running, walking, and hiking. This type of exercise helps to build muscle and strengthen bones.

Resources

American College of Obstetrics and Gynecology. "Exercise During Pregnancy and the Postpartum Period." Committee Opinion Number 267. *American Journal of Obstetrics and Gynecology* 99, no. 1 (January 2002), 171–73.

"Exercise During Pregnancy and the Postpartum Period." Technical Bulletin Number 189. *International Journal of Gynecology and Obstetrics* 45, no. 1 (April 1994), 65–70.

"Assessment of Risk Factors for Preterm Birth." Committee Opinion Number 251. *Obstetrics and Gynecology* 98, no. 4 (October 2001), 709–16.

Beister, E., et al. "Trauma in Pregnancy: Normal Revised Trauma Score in Relation to Other Markers of Maternofetal Status—a Preliminary Study." *American Journal of Obstetrics and Gynecology* 176 (1997), 1206–212.

Bell, R., et al. "Exercise and Pregnancy: a Review." *Birth* 21, no. 2 (1994), 85–95.

Bo, K., T. Talseth, and I. Holme. "Single Blind, Randomised Controlled Trial of Pelvic Floor Exercises, Electrical Stimulation, Vaginal Cones, and No Treatment in Management of Genuine Stress Incontinence in Women." *British Medical Journal* 318, no. 7182 (1999), 487–93.

Camporesi, E. "Diving and Pregnancy." *Seminars in Perinatology* 20, no. 4 (1996), 292–302.

Carey, G. B., T. J. Quinn, and S. E. Goodwin. "Breast Milk Composition After Exercise of Different Intensities." *Journal of Human Lactation* 13, no. 2 (1997), 115–20.

Centers for Disease Control and Prevention. National Center for Infectious Diseases. http://www.cdc.gov/travel/bugs.htm.

Clapp, J. "Exercise and Fetal Health." *Journal of Developmental Physiology* 15 (1991), 9–14.

"Exercise During Pregnancy: A Clinical Update." *Clinics in Sports Medicine* 19, no. 2 (April 2000), 273–86.

"The Course of Labor After Endurance Exercise During Pregnancy." *American Journal of Obstetrics and Gynecology* 163 (1990), 1799–804.

"Pregnancy Outcome: Physical Activities Inside Versus Outside the Workplace." *Seminars in Perinatology* 20 (January 1996), 70–76.

"A Clinical Approach to Exercise During Pregnancy." *Clinics in Sports Medicine* 13, no. 2 (1994), 443–57.

"The Morphometric and Neurodeveopmental Outcome at Five Years of the Offspring of Women Who Continued to Exercise Throughout Pregnancy. *Journal of Pediatrics* 129 (1996), 856–63.

Clapp, J., et al. "The Changing Glycemic Response to Exercise During Pregnancy." *American Journal of Obstetrics and Gynecology* 165 (1991), 1678–83.

Clapp, J., et al. "Thermoregulatory and Metabolic Responses to Jogging Prior to and During Pregnancy." *Medicine and Science in Sports and Exercise* 19 (1987), 124–30.

Clapp, J., et al. "Neonatal Behavioral Profile of the Offspring of Women Who Continued to Exercise Regularly Throughout Pregnancy." *American Journal of Obstetrics and Gynecology* 180, no. 1 (January 1999), 91–94.

Crowell, D. T. "Weight Change in the Postpartum Period: A Review of the Literature." *Journal of Nurse Midwifery* 40, no. 5 (1995), 418–23.

Elia, G. "Stress Urinary Incontinence in Women: Removing the Barriers to Exercise." *The Physician and Sportsmedicine* 27, no. 1 (1999), 39–52.

Fildes, J., et al. "Trauma: The Leading Cause of Maternal Death." *Journal of Trauma* 32 (1992), 643–45.

Hackett, P. "High Altitude and Common Medical Conditions." In *High Altitude: An Exploration of Human Adaptation.* New York: Dekker, 2001.

Hale, R. W. "The Elite Athlete and Exercise in Pregnancy." *Seminars in Perinatology* 20, no. 4 (1996), 277–84.

Hall, D. C. "Effects of Aerobic Strength and Conditioning on Pregnancy Outcomes." *American Journal of Obstetrics and Gynecology* 157 (1987), 1199–203.

Hartmann, S., et al. "Physical Exercise During Pregnancy: Physiological Considerations and Recommendations." *Journal of Perinatal Medicine* 27, no. 3 (1999), 204–15.

Hatch, C. M., et al. "Maternal Exercise During Pregnancy, Physical Fitness, and Fetal Growth." *American Journal of Epidemiology* 137 (1993), 1105–14.

Jackson, M., et al. "The Effects of Maternal Aerobic Exercise on Human Placental Development: Placental Volumetric Composition and Surface Areas." *Placenta* 16 (1995), 179–91.

Jarrett, J. C., et al. "Jogging During Pregnancy: An Improved Outcome?" *Obstetrics and Gynecology* 16 (1984), 705–9.

Katz, V. "Water Exercise in Pregnancy." *Seminars in Perinatology* 20, no. 4 (August 1996), 285–91.

Keppel, K. G., and S. M. Taffel. "Pregnancy-Related Weight Gain and Retention: Implications of the 1990 Institute of Medicine Guidelines." *American Journal of Public Health* 83, no. 8 (1993), 1100–1103.

Lederman, S. A. "The Effect of Pregnancy Weight Gain on Later Obesity." *Obstetrics and Gynecology* 82, no. 1 (1993), 148–55.

Little, K. D., et al. "Effect of Recreational Exercise on Pregnancy Weight Gain and Subcutaneous Fat Deposition." *Medicine and Science in Sports and Exercise* 27 (1995), 170–77.

Little, K. D., et al. "Effect of Exercise on Postpartum Weight and Subcutaneous Fat Loss." *Medicine and Science in Sports and Exercise* 26 (1994), 14.

Lokey, E. A., et al. "Effect of Physical Exercise on Pregnancy Outcomes: A Meta-Analytic Review." *Medicine and Science in Sports and Exercise* 23 (1991), 1234–39.

McCormick, R. D. "Seat Belt Injury: Case of Complete Transection of Pregnant Uterus." *Journal of the American Osteopathic Association* 67 (1968), 1139–41.

McCrory, M. A., L. A. Nommsen-Rivers, P. A. Molé, et al. "Randomized Trial of the Short-Term Effects of Dieting Compared with Dieting plus Aerobic Exercise on Lactation Performance." *American Journal of Clinical Nutrition* 69, no. 5 (1999), 959–67.

Meyers, J. P. "From Silent Spring to Scientific Revolution." *San Francisco Medicine* (November 2002).

Nygaard, I. E., J. O. DeLancey, L. Arnsdorf, et al. "Exercise and Incontinence." *Obstetrics and Gynecology* 75, no. 5 (1990), 848–51.

Nygaard, I. E., F. L. Thompson, S. L. Svengalis, et al. "Urinary Incontinence in Elite Nulliparous Athletes." *Obstetrics and Gynecology* 84, no. 2 (1994), 183–87.

Ostgaard, H. C., et al. "Reduction of Back and Posterior Pelvic Pain in Pregnancy." *Spine* 19 (1994), 894–900.

Perlman, M. D., and D. Viano. "Automobile Crash Simulation with the First Pregnant Crash Test Dummy." *American Journal of Obstetrics and Gynecology* 175 (1996), 977–81.

Pivarnik, J. M., N. A. Ayre, M. B. Mauer, et al. "Effects of Maternal Aerobic Fitness on Cardio-Respiratory Responses to Exercise." *Medicine and Science in Sports and Exercise* 25, no. 9 (September 1993), 993–98.

Pivarnik, J. M, et al. "Effect of Chronic Exercise on Blood Volume Expansion and Hematologic Indices During Pregnancy." *Obstetrics and Gynecology* 83 (1994), 265–69.

Pivarnik, J. M., et al. "Cardiac Output Responses of Primigravid Women during Exercise Determined by the Direct Fick Technique." *Obstetrics and Gynecology* 75 (1990), 954–59.

Pivarnik, J. M., et al. "Maternal Respiration and Blood Gases During Aerobic Exercise Performed at Moderate Altitude." *Medicine and Science in Sports and Exercise* 24 (1992), 868–72.

Quinn, T. J., and G. B. Carey. "Is Breast Milk Composition in Lactating Women Altered by Exercise Intensity or Diet?" *Medicine and Science in Sports and Exercise* 29 (1997), S4.

Rabkin, C. S., et al. "Maternal Activity and Birth Weight: A Prospective Population-Based Study." *American Journal of Epidemiology* 131 (1990), 522–31.

Robson, S. C., et al. "Serial Study of Factors Influencing Changes in Cardiac Output During Human Pregnancy." *American Journal of Physiology* 256 (1989), H1060–H1065.

Sowers, M., M. Crutchfield, M. Jannausch, et al. "A Prospective Evaluation of Bone Mineral Change in Pregnancy." *Obstetrics and Gynecology* 77 (1991), 841–45.

Wallace, J. P., G. Inbar, and K. Ernsthausen. "Lactate Concentrations in Breast Milk Following Maximal Exercise and a Typical Workout." *Journal of Women's Health* 3, no. 2 (1994), 91–96.

"Infant Acceptance of Post-Exercise Breast Milk." *Pediatrics* 89 (1992), 1245–47.

Wang, T., et al. "Exercise During Pregnancy." *American Family Physician* 57, no. 8 (1998), 1846–52.

Wolfe, L. A., et al. "Effects of Pregnancy and Chronic Exercise on Respiratory Responses to Graded Exercises." *Journal of Applied Physiology* 76 (1994), 1928–36.

Wong, S. C., and D. C. McKenzie. "Cardiorespiratory Fitness During Pregnancy and Its Effects on Outcome." *International Journal of Sports Medicine* 8 (1987), 79–83.

Index